HOW TO COPE
SUCCESSFULLY WITH

HIGH CHOLESTEROL

DR TOM SMITH

Wellhouse Publishing Ltd

First published in Great Britain in 2002 by
Wellhouse Publishing Ltd
31 Middle Bourne Lane
Lower Bourne
Farnham
Surrey GU10 3NH

Dr Tom Smith asserts the moral right to be
identified as the author of this work.

DISCLAIMER

The aim of this book is to provide general information only and should not be treated as a substitute for the medical advice of your doctor or any other health care professional. The publisher and author is not responsible or liable for any diagnosis made by a reader based on the contents of this book. Always consult your doctor if you are in any way concerned about your health.

A catalogue record for this book is available from the British Library

ISBN 1 903784 09 3

Printed and bound in Great Britain by
Biddles Ltd., Surrey. www.biddles.co.uk

Contents

For my fellow graduates of 1962 from
Birmingham Medical School.

They could not have been better friends
over the last 40 years.

Introduction

It seems a long time since we were all exhorted to 'go to work on an egg' and to 'drink a pint of milk a day.' These two messages, so popular in the 1960s, fell out of favour in the 1970s. That was when cholesterol raised its ugly head, and eggs and dairy products were transformed into foods that would harm, rather than help, your heart. The messages changed to 'eat only three eggs a week' and 'have the odd drink of semi-skimmed milk from time to time.' We were all encouraged to have our blood cholesterol levels checked regularly, and to eat foods that would keep them down, or at least to reasonable levels.

Why did these messages change so drastically? Were the people who changed the messages right? What is cholesterol, anyway? Should we be worried about it, and its level in our blood? Does changing what we eat really make much difference? Does bringing down blood cholesterol really lower our risk of a heart attack or stroke? Do the drugs so many of us take really make a difference? Are there other things we should be doing as well, to make an even bigger difference to our chances of having a heart attack or stroke?

This book aims to answer these questions and more. It is about cholesterol and the related fatty substances, called *lipids*, which have been identified as important in causing heart disease and strokes. It explains why we have lipids in our bloodstream and tissues, what they do, why sometimes we need to take notice of them, and what we can do – by eating wisely, exercising and making other lifestyle changes – to lessen the havoc they may wreak on our blood vessels. If we can do that we stand a better chance of avoiding an early death from heart attack or stroke.

Other Causes of Heart Attacks and Strokes

Cholesterol and the other blood lipids are only a small part of the story of heart disease, however. On its own, a higher-than-normal level of cholesterol in your blood doesn't normally pose much of a risk. There are exceptions: a very few men and women inherit a tendency to develop extremely high cholesterol levels. For them it is vital that everything should be done, including permanently taking drugs, to lower these levels, and we shall discuss this later in the book. For the vast majority, however, what is called for is a broader approach to a healthier life and to lowering their risks of heart attack and strokes, which may or may not involve drugs.

Doctors have known for at least 20 years that there are three main 'risk factors' promoting heart attacks and strokes:

1. Uncontrolled high blood pressure, or *hypertension*.
2. Smoking
3. A high blood lipid level.
   The medical term for a high blood fat (lipid) level is *hyperlipidaemia*, but it is so closely linked to blood cholesterol levels in the popular press that it is usually referred to as 'a high cholesterol'.
   There are two other 'secondary' risk factors that promote heart attacks and strokes:
4. Obesity
5. A sedentary lifestyle

Obviously these last two are linked: People who take little exercise tend to be overweight. But the two are not always found together. There are slim couch potatoes, presumably because they don't eat much (although these people are rare). And there are people who take plenty of exercise but also eat a lot. Weight-lifters and sumo wrestlers come to mind.

There is one more risk factor which applies to more and more men and women in their middle years and beyond. That is maturity-onset diabetes. The recent figures for this illness are worrying: it affects more than two million people in Britain, and the numbers are rising steeply, year on year.

This book, therefore, not only covers cholesterol but has specific chapters on high blood pressure, smoking, exercise, body shape and diabetes. They all matter to men and women who have been told they have a high cholesterol.

It cannot be emphasised enough that you mustn't look at your cholesterol levels in isolation: they are part of a whole series of problems. There is a chapter on the drugs used to treat high cholesterol levels, but please don't buy the book just to read about them. If you do, and you ignore the rest of the lifestyle advice, you will be doing yourself a disservice.

I'm not in favour of buzz words like 'holistic' in medicine. I believe that all general practitioners like myself, who take pride in their work, treat the 'whole patient'. We practised holistically before the word was hijacked by complementary and alternative practitioners. But if the word holistic has any meaning at all, it is in the treatment of people with a high cholesterol level. You ignore a high cholesterol at your peril, but if you do the opposite, and concentrate on it alone, you are making just as big a mistake. Take all the advice in this book together, as a complete guide to your future good health.

Chapter One

Your Least-known Organ – The Endothelium

Crucial to why cholesterol is so important is an understanding of the least-known organ in the body. Ask people to name the main organs of the body and they will mention the brain, the heart, the liver, the lungs, the kidneys, then maybe start to flounder a bit. They might add the pancreas or the gut, or the uterus or prostate, but that's all. A few may consider, correctly, that the skin is an organ.

All these organs have in common that they are very specialised tissues with very particular functions. The brain provides us with the ability to think, to sense the environment around us, and to react to it. The heart pumps blood around the body. The liver deals with food and its conversion into the essential substances for our daily living. The lungs give us oxygen and expel waste carbon dioxide and water. The kidneys get rid of waste fluids. The pancreas organises our blood glucose levels and produces digestive enzymes. The skin controls our body temperature and protects us against infection, among other things.

So far, you probably haven't read anything that you don't already know about organs from your school biology classes. But there is another organ, at least as important as all the others, that hardly anyone outside medicine knows about. In a normal 70-kilogram human, this organ, spread out, would cover the surface of six tennis courts. It is easily the largest organ in the body, weighing more than the liver, yet no pathologist has ever been able to weigh it. The cells in it alone number around 1,000,000,000,000.

The Endothelium

This amazing organ is the *endothelium*. It is the single layer of cells that lines every blood vessel in your body – in effect the 'inside skin' of your arteries and veins. Much of what we know about it stems from the work of Professor Howard Florey. Professor Florey was one of the pioneers in the development of penicillin in the 1940s, work for which he is rightly remembered and highly esteemed. But I would argue that his discovery of what the endothelium does is even more important. Working on it in the 1950s, with few of today's technical advantages, Howard Florey showed how a healthy endothelium was fundamental in controlling how substances flow from the bloodstream into the tissues and vice versa.

Before his work, it was assumed that the endothelium acted as both a barrier and a filter. It allowed, so the theory went, essential substances like fats, proteins and glucose, vitamins and minerals to pass through it from the bloodstream into the tissues, while being an impenetrable barrier to more solid substances like white and red blood cells and bacteria. At the same time, back out from the tissues through the endothelium into the bloodstream would come waste products from the breakdown of foodstuffs, like urea, the basis of urine. Otherwise, the theory went, the endothelium was a fairly passive structure.

Howard Florey proved that this was far too simplistic. The electron microscope, new in the 1950s, showed him the detailed structure of the cells and, just as important, the gaps between them, in the endothelium. He described for the first time how large molecules, like proteins and complex fats, and even large structures like certain white blood cells, could pass through and between the endothelial cells. He also hinted at discoveries to come of the vast number of ways in which the cells actively promote the passage, in both directions, of the body's huge numbers of biochemical 'messenger' substances essential to the process of living.

Thanks to Florey, we now know that the endothelium not only transports these substances in either direction between blood and tissues, but is also very active in manufacturing them. In effect, it is at least as important in controlling major functions of the body as are organs like the pancreas and the liver. The endothelium is vital to the normal regulation of blood pressure, of our fluid and mineral balance and, most important for the subject of this book, the distribution and deposition of fats into our tissues. When healthy, the cells in the endothelium are extremely sensitive to changes in the chemistry, flow and pressure of the blood inside it. When it becomes unhealthy, and less responsive, all these processes start to go awry.

What the Endothelium Does for Us

I'll give an example without being too technical. Blood vessels are hollow tubes with layers of linings around them. The first, innermost, lining is the endothelium, that single-cell layer which Howard Florey studied. Immediately around it is a layer of 'connective tissue', a loose network, or mesh, of cells and elastic fibres which provide physical and chemical support for the endothelium. And around that is a muscle layer, the contraction and relaxation of which control the 'bore' of the tube through which the blood flows. Cause the muscles to contract, and you narrow the bore. That means the heart must work harder to push the blood through it, and your blood pressure rises.

To counteract this, the endothelium releases substances to relax the muscles, which widen the bore again, the flow increases, and the pressure falls. So a healthy endothelium is essential to the control of blood pressure – an unhealthy endothelium which doesn't release the right muscle-relaxing substances can contribute to high blood pressure. That can be the first step to a heart attack or stroke.

This single property of the endothelium is only the start. Since Howard Florey's time we have found that the endothelium responds vigorously to all sorts of abnormalities in the blood – such as too low an oxygen content, or shock from blood loss due to injury, or toxins from infections. It responds in an extremely complex way to injury, producing substances that control blood clotting and sending messages to the healing white cells to travel to the scene of the injury or infection. If part of the endothelium is injured, it quickly lays down a new layer of cells to carry on its work of control and healing. It releases hormones into the blood that are detected by the kidneys, which respond by altering the body's fluid balance appropriately. It measures the amounts of fats and glucose in the blood, and controls their transport from the bloodstream into the tissues accordingly.

The endothelium also combats diseases. If there are substances in the bloodstream that are 'foreign' to the body, such as germs and their chemical by-products, the endothelium will detect them and organise the body's defences against them. This may mean marshalling white blood cells to the spot, or initiating the process of producing 'antibodies' – chemical substances specifically formed to attach themselves to the surface of germs and their products.

By now you will have realised that the endothelium is a pretty important organ. Anything you may do to keep it healthy is good for you. Anything you do to harm it or stop it from working at full capacity is obviously bad for you.

Cholesterol and the Endothelium

This is where we have to start thinking about cholesterol and what it can do to the endothelium. The story starts with the Korean War, in the 1950s. At that time doctors were beginning to worry about what appeared to be an epidemic of heart disease among middle-aged Americans. As the country had become more affluent, the numbers of Americans in their forties and older who were dropping dead or being severely disabled from heart attacks had been rising steeply. The researchers wanted to know why this was happening, and what processes were occurring in the arteries – and particularly the coronary arteries bringing oxygenated blood from the lungs to the heart muscle – that were causing them to block and fail.

One of the research projects was a particularly grisly one. It was to perform post-mortem examinations on young American servicemen who had been killed in action. Sadly there were plenty of subjects aged around 20 years old. All had been passed as perfectly fit to be sent to the front line. The pathologists were astounded to find that they were all showing signs of early fatty degeneration in the walls of their arteries. Instead of the smooth, red, unblemished endothelium that they expected, there were many rough areas under which could be seen yellow streaks of fatty material. The main problems were in the aorta, the major artery leading from the heart to the rest of the body, but in many of the young men the coronary arteries were also already affected by the same process.

The researchers concluded that these 'fatty streaks' were the start of the process that would have eventually led to deaths from heart disease and strokes if the young men had not been killed in battle. That conclusion was taken very seriously, and was the impetus for the American authorities, academics in medical schools, and the pharmaceutical industry to invest billions of dollars in research into arterial disease.

Curiously, we now believe that the fatty streaks are probably not what they seemed to be. Over the years it has turned out that they are probably a normal aspect of artery wall structure, and not necessarily a portent of disaster to come. Only a minority of people with them go on to develop severe fatty degeneration of their arteries, and therefore heart attacks and strokes. So, researchers have turned to the study of the next stage of arterial disease – the *atheromatous plaque*. If you have a high cholesterol, it is very much worthwhile spending some time learning about this, because it is the key to your survival in good health.

Atheroma

Atheroma comes from the ancient Greek word for 'porridge'. Plaques (tiny patches) of atheroma in the lining of your arteries have the grey appearance and consistency of porridge, hence the name. Examine the arteries of people in their forties and older, and many of them will show such patches, particularly in the arteries of the heart and brain. In those who have died from heart attacks and strokes, it is often evident that a plaque has been the site of a clot or a tear that has led to a block in, or a bleed from, a vital artery. Clots and bleeds are the causes of heart attacks and strokes.

Atheromatous plaques are complex structures. They are made up of accumulations of solidified fats, interspersed with aggregates of the remains of white blood cells and platelets. Platelets are tiny particles, smaller than white blood cells, that are normally present in the bloodstream. They initiate clotting by sticking together and to any injured surface in the endothelium. Within and under the plaques are also what can best be described as a network of fibres, in effect scar tissue that has been deposited there as a reaction to inflammation.

On the outer surface of each plaque lies a layer of muscle. However, it is not normal muscle. It is usually much thicker than normal, because the muscle cells at the site have 'proliferated', or overgrown. The overall result is that, at the site of a plaque, the channel through which the blood is meant to flow is narrowed by the bulging and thickened wall (see diagram). Instead of a smooth flow of blood within the artery, it is buffeted by passing over the roughened and narrowed area. There may even be eddy currents in the blood at that point.

Narrowing of the flow, and turbulence within it, can lead to a vicious cycle in the artery. With less blood flowing through the narrowed artery, less oxygen is getting to the tissues beyond. With turbulent flow there is mechanical strain on the artery wall, and that can lead to tears and the deposition of clots on the ragged surface.

The endothelium over the surface of a plaque no longer works efficiently. It no longer produces the chemicals that tell the muscles (which are already overdeveloped and prone to contract) to relax, nor the chemicals that signal the need for healing white cells and proteins. Further clotting and narrowing damages the arterial wall further, until it breaks down completely and either gives way in a bleed or develops a blockage.

Diagram 1: A Plaque in an Artery

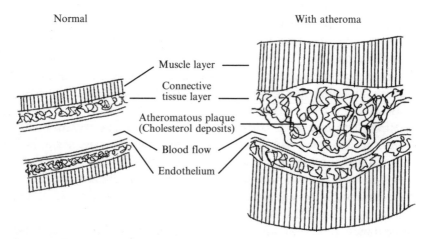

The Role Cholesterol Plays

The higher your blood cholesterol level, the more fat will be deposited just under the endothelium, in the connective tissue layer, in the walls of your arteries. If that is allowed to continue, more plaques will form. The more plaques in your arteries, the higher is your chance of having a heart attack and/or stroke. It is as simple as that. *Lower your cholesterol level and you will substantially lower that chance.* If there is one message to be learned from this book, that is it.

But don't depend on lowering cholesterol alone. You must also tackle other aspects of your life that harm your endothelium. If you have high blood pressure that is not well controlled, then those muscles wrapped round your arteries will grow thicker, and narrow your arteries, making a blockage much more likely. It will also put extra strain on areas of plaque, so that they can split asunder, tear the artery wall, and cause a bleed. In the brain this is known as a 'haemorrhagic' stroke.

If you smoke, then you directly damage your endothelium with each inhalation. The thousand or so damaging chemicals in smoke pass into your blood and poison that very delicate single layer of cells that lines every artery. Smokers have very many fewer functioning endothelial cells than non-smokers. This leads to many problems for the circulation. For a start, the endothelium cannot give the signal to the muscle layer to relax, so that the calibre of the tube through which the blood has to flow is greatly reduced. That means less oxygen getting through to the tissues beyond. In fact, smoking already compromises the oxygen supply to the artery wall because so many of smokers' red cells carry carbon monoxide, rather than oxygen, around the body. And you can't use carbon monoxide for energy! It is a deadly poison.

Smoking also harms the arteries by promoting blood-clotting. It increases the blood levels of a substance, fibrinogen, that is the most powerful natural blood-clotting agent. It also makes the platelets much more active, so that they stick to the artery walls and to each other far more easily – and once stuck together, they stay stuck.

And then there is nicotine. Smokers of even one cigarette a day put enough nicotine in their blood to cause the muscles around the arteries to contract – making the arteries, already under an onslaught, even narrower. If you were deliberately to try to design a drug that would kill people with a heart attack or stroke, you could not possibly do better than tobacco.

Finally, if you have diabetes, constantly higher than normal levels of glucose in your blood, along with high blood pressure, can also damage the endothelium. So do follow your strict plan of diabetes and blood pressure control.

The message of this chapter, therefore, is to look on your endothelium in the same way as you look on your brain, your lungs, your heart and your liver. Most of us dread the thought of our brain going in old age, and ending up with dementia. So we try to stave it off by keeping it active. We know about our lungs, and how smoking affects them. We all know of the messages about a healthy heart – no one could have missed the promotion of healthy eating, such as five portions of fruit and vegetables a day, with oily fish and perhaps red wine thrown in. We all know that excess drinking harms our liver. But how many of us know that we need to look after our endothelium, too? And how important cholesterol and other fats in our blood are to keeping it healthy?

Keeping the endothelium healthy is the key to keeping all the other organs healthy, too. There is endothelium in the brain, heart, lungs and liver, and looking after it will protect them all.

To understand the role of blood lipids like cholesterol in protecting the endothelium, we need to know more about the 'good' and 'bad' lipids, how they come to be in the blood at all, and what they do. That is the subject of Chapter Two.

Chapter Two

Cholesterol and Other Blood Lipids

Perhaps you are wondering why we have cholesterol in the blood at all, considering that it does so much damage to our arteries? I can best answer that by posing a 'pub quiz'- type question. What is the fattest organ in the body? In other words, the one that contains the highest proportion of fat (in comparison with protein or glucose)?

The answer is the brain.

The brain needs a lot of fat, because fat is an essential component of nerve cells and their 'insulating' covering, a substance called *myelin*. Without myelin separating nerve cell fibres from each other, the electrical signal that runs along the fibres would dissipate into the surrounding tissues, and the nervous system would not work. This is, in fact, the problem in people with multiple sclerosis: their myelin sheaths deteriorate, and their nerves fail to work.

So we need to transport fats around our bodies to keep our organs healthy and working to maximum capacity. We do that by using the 'family' of fats, one group of which is cholesterol-based.

Fatty Acids

Cholesterol has a complex chemical structure, the details of which are outside the remit of this book. It is enough to state that its 'building blocks' are derived from fatty acids that we obtain in the first place from fat in our food. The story goes like this. We swallow food containing fat or oil. As it hits the stomach, it sends a chemical message to the liver to squirt some bile via a tube, the bile duct, into the duodenum, the section of gut that lies just beyond the stomach. The bile mixes with the fat from the food in the duodenum and starts the process of digestion. The end-product of that digestion is a series of fatty acids, which are taken up through the gut wall into the bloodstream, and from there into the liver.

The liver cells can be likened to a factory turning the fatty acids into two substances – cholesterol and bile. The bile is passed back into the gut, to digest the next load of fat from the food. The cholesterol is passed into the bloodstream, where it is transported into the tissues that need it, and is converted into the type of fat that that particular organ needs. For example, it can be myelin for nerve tissue, or 'phospholipids' (fats attached to phosphate molecules) or 'lipoproteins' (fats combined with proteins) for specialist jobs in brain and nerve cells, or for breast milk, or converted into simpler fats for storage around our gut or under the skin.

Why Do We Need to Store Fat?

To answer this we need to digress for a while into human history. Fat storage is a relic from our hundreds of thousands of years as hunter-gatherers, when we had to face many times of near-famine. We ate as much as we could in times of plenty so that we could live on our fat stores in times of near-starvation. Our usual immediate source of energy is glucose, which we make in our gut from the digestion of sugars and starches, but we have very limited capacity to store it. In fact, glucose is stored as a substance called glycogen in some muscles and the liver, but all our body's supply of glycogen can quickly be used up when we exert ourselves. From then on we have to use stored fats as our energy source.

We inherited from our Stone Age ancestors a very efficient system for storing fats, so that they can be used as fuel for our muscles, brain and other organs when we have nothing to eat or have used up our glucose and glycogen. Conditions ten thousand years ago or more probably kept our ancestors thin, as they would use up all the fat they could consume in their daily lives. Today, everyone in developed societies has enough to eat. If we do not use up all the fat and glucose we eat each day in energetic activity, then we have to store it, and almost all of it is stored as fat. Even with normal body shapes, with no obesity, the average woman is 18 per cent, and the average man 10 per cent, fat.

However, fewer and fewer of us have normal body shapes. We exercise far less than we used to, and we eat and drink more. Today, by the time we reach 50, nearly half of us, men and women alike, are overweight enough to be described as obese. That means at least 30 per cent fat, and perhaps a lot more.

Where Does the Fat Go?

The answer to this is crucial for every reader of this book. We may put it on our waists, our hips, our backs (in a 'buffalo hump'), or space it fairly equally under the skin all round our torso and limbs. It is also laid down in the walls of our arteries, as streaks and plaques just under the endothelium. Classically, people are described as 'apples' (with fat mainly around the waist and inside the abdomen) or 'pears' (with most of the fat around the hips and bottom). There is some evidence that apples are more prone to heart attacks than pears, because they lay more fat in their artery walls than the pears do – but any form of obesity raises our risk.

However, the message of this chapter isn't just about obesity. There are some (not many) obese people with relatively low 'bad' cholesterol levels in their blood, and there are thin people (again, not many) who have high 'bad' cholesterol levels. And of the two, those with the high cholesterol levels, whether they are fat or thin, are more likely to have a heart attack or stroke.

'Good' and 'Bad' Cholesterol

When doctors first began to take note of blood cholesterol levels years ago, all they did was to measure 'total cholesterol' and treat people on the basis that, if high, it had to be brought down.

Now, in the light of further research, we are far more sophisticated. It is not acceptable just to rely on total cholesterol levels. We need to know about the different types of cholesterol and other fats (lipids) in the blood, and decide on what to do accordingly. The next few paragraphs summarise what we know about the different forms of blood lipids – the ones you will see on your lab report when your doctor discusses your treatment with you.

Sorting Out the Fats

First let's have some definitions. The medical name for fat of any sort is *lipid*. 'Blood lipid level' is the term for the amount of fats in your venous blood, taken usually from a vein in your arm. The lipids we are most concerned about fall into two main categories: cholesterol and triglyceride. However, they don't float about in the blood on their own. Most molecules of cholesterol and triglyceride in the blood are transported around attached to proteins, so they are called 'lipoprotein complexes'. The different types of lipoprotein complex are identified by spinning the plasma (blood from which the red cells have been removed) in a centrifuge. That separates out the different lipoproteins from each other according to how dense (heavy) they are. So there are very low-density lipoproteins (VLDLs), low-density lipoproteins (LDLs), and high-density lipoproteins (HDLs). Triglyceride is usually carried in VLDLs, and cholesterol in LDLs or HDLs. So in your blood test report, TC means total cholesterol, and LDL-C, VLDL-C and HDL-C refer to the various types of cholesterol levels. TG stands for triglyceride level. It's important not to confuse TC with TG.

Generally speaking, LDLs are considered 'bad' cholesterol, while HDLs are considered 'good'. More about this later on.

Some cholesterol and triglyceride does remain unattached to proteins and remains as free lipid in the blood, but in healthy people this is relatively unimportant. The body attaches fats to proteins (to form lipoproteins) because this is the only way in which lipids can be transported across the healthy endothelium – in either direction. Combined with protein, the fat molecule is soluble, and is easy for the endothelium to handle. As a free fat in the blood, either as cholesterol or triglyceride, it remains relatively insoluble, cannot cross the intact endothelium, and remains in the blood. However, if the endothelium is damaged, it is a different story. Without an intact layer of healthy endothelial cells to protect the blood vessel wall, the fats and triglyceride can pass into the wall, where they are laid down as solid deposits, helping to form the structure of plaques.

Your blood test result will probably indicate your levels of triglyceride, HDL and LDL, along with your total cholesterol. If that is not enough to worry about, you may also be shown your levels of apolipoproteins, a family of lipid-protein complexes that have been divided into five main groups, from A to E. All that we need to know about the apolipoproteins here is that LDL contains mainly apo-B, and HDL mainly apo-A lipoproteins.

How Does This Relate to Heart Disease and Strokes?

Local hospital laboratories all over the world measure blood lipid levels in their own populations, and relate the results in each individual to this normal range. The normal range differs from country to country, within areas of the same country, and even within populations of different districts in the same city. So it is difficult to be precise in a book like this on what is 'normal' and what is 'high' for you.

However, specialists in vascular diseases (diseases of the blood vessels) and in metabolic diseases (which includes lipid disorders) have defined what they see as acceptable generally for everyone. Everyone with lipid levels (often called a 'lipid profile') likely to cause concern is given a general diagnosis of *dyslipidaemia*. The term simply means abnormal levels of fat in the blood.

If you have a higher-than-normal level of TC or LDL-C, this is called *hypercholesterolaemia* (*hyper* means 'too much'; *aemia* means 'in the blood'). Too high a TG level is called *hypertriglyceridaemia*, and when both cholesterol and TG are raised, it is called *combined hyperlipidaemia*.

Some people have low HDL-C levels, but their other lipids are in the normal range: they are diagnosed as having *dyslipidaemia*. However, a low HDL-C almost always goes with hypertriglyceridaemia, so low HDL-C on its own is relatively rare. All these types of dyslipidaemia may be inborn (inherited with your genes), 'secondary' (brought on by lifestyle), or a combination of both.

Crucial to the recognition of dyslipidaemias is that they are very strongly related to your risk of having heart attacks and strokes. In particular, the worse your hypercholesterolaemia or hypertriglyceridaemia, or both, the higher is your risk of succumbing to one of these catastrophes. The risk rises throughout the range of blood cholesterol, from the lowest of all to the highest, and the slope is a steep one.

We measure lipid levels in Britain in millimoles of each type of lipid per litre (mmol/l) of blood. In the United States, they are measured in milligrams per decilitre (mg/dl) of blood. As 1mmol/l cholesterol is the equivalent of 38.68mg/dl, if you are in the American health system, multiply the mmol/l figures given in this book by 40 and you will have a good idea of your own risks.

A man with a total plasma cholesterol (TC) level of 5.2mmol/l has half the risk of coronary heart disease (angina and heart attack) of one with a TC of 6.5mmol/l, and only a quarter of the risk of a man with a TC of 7.8mmol/l. Put another way, if you reduce your TC from 7.8 to 5.2 you will reduce your heart attack risk by three quarters.

This is not guesswork. It has been proved time and time again in populations within countries and in comparisons between countries. Countries with low TC levels like Japan (average around 4.9mmol/l) have about 60 deaths per 100,000 people per year: in those with averages above 6mmol/l, like my own country, Scotland, the corresponding figure is 600. Finland used to have similar figures – 10 times those of the Japanese – but since its government initiated a huge healthy lifestyle campaign both the TC levels and the numbers of deaths have plummeted.

The relationship between TC levels and deaths from heart attacks is constant for almost every country. Take Poland, with a TC average of 5.5 and a death rate of 280, or Germany, with 5.7 and 320, and England with 6.5 and 470. One exception is France, with an average TC of 5.8 and a death rate of only 135. That is almost certainly explained by the regular consumption in France of red wine, about which there is more later.

However, a rise in TC alone does not explain all the cholesterol-related deaths. When concerns were raised in the 1950s about the steep increase in heart disease, health experts all over the world started to study their own populations 'prospectively'. That is, they selected healthy people for close follow-up over many years, having first measured their blood lipid profiles. Some were left to follow their usual lifestyles without interference, other trials promoted what was thought then to be a healthier lifestyle for hearts to some subjects and not to others. The goal was to follow as many as possible to their eventual deaths, and to record their age at death and the cause.

Trial Results

The results of most of these trials were published in the 1980s, and they became the basis for almost all we do to manage high blood lipid levels today. Certainly they provided the motivation to doctors to ensure that their patients should keep their lipid profiles as healthy as possible. The different studies are described in more detail in the next chapter, so it is enough here to give the general conclusions.

All the studies confirmed that men with higher TC levels were more likely to die from heart attacks and strokes than those with lower TC levels. But in each study there were substantial numbers of men with low TC levels who still died early. This was true in countries in continental Europe, the United States and the United Kingdom. In the

British Regional Heart Study,[1] one in five of the men recorded as having serious or fatal heart attacks or strokes had TCs below 6mmol/l. They were in the lowest 40 per cent of the range of TC results.

Why did so many people with relatively low TCs die? There are several ways of explaining this. Perhaps a TC of 6mmol/l is still far too high for safety. It is certainly very much higher than the average Japanese TC. We should probably aim for a TC under 5mmol/l. Or there may be other aspects of their lipids, such as a high TG and LDL-C, with a low HDL-C, that were not measured in the studies. Or other factors, such as high blood pressure, smoking habits and diabetes, may have played their part.

In fact, all these explanations are true. High blood pressure, smoking and diabetes will be discussed in later chapters, but this is the place to discuss the other lipids.

How Are Fats Deposited into the Endothelium?

Why should some lipids, like LDL-C and TG, be thought to be 'bad' for us, and HDL-C be thought to be 'good'? Let's go back to the idea of fats being deposited into the endothelium, where they cause plaques of atheroma, and eventually block or rupture the artery. The most recent view of how this happens is that the liver receives fatty acids, as described earlier, from the bowel after our digestion forms them by breaking down fats in our food. The liver cells then start the process of turning the fatty acids into triglyceride and cholesterol. The combination of the two with protein forms VLDL-C. This is the most suitable form of fat for release from the liver into the bloodstream. Once there, it is then ready for delivery to the smallest blood vessels for transport across the endothelium into the tissues. On the way, the VLDL-C is progressively enriched with more cholesterol, which makes the molecules more dense – forming LDL-C. The endothelium is therefore faced with VLDL-C and LDL-C, which it must carry across into the tissues beyond, so that the fat can be used for the building and energy processes described earlier.

So far, so good. But what happens if there is too much VLDL-C and LDL-C? Some of it circulates back to the liver, where it is taken up by the liver cells and stored for future use. Some of it is taken up by fat - storage cells. But a sizeable proportion of it remains in the connective tissue layer just beyond the endothelium, where it is treated by the body as an irritant, and 'scavenged' by white blood cells called to the site to deal with it. The white cells fill with cholesterol and become 'foam' cells, so named because under the microscope they look as if they are filled with foam.

Foam cells do not survive long. They die, releasing free cholesterol into the artery wall. If this state continues, platelets are attracted to the area, and form tiny 'thromboses' on the surface. This is the beginning of a plaque. High VLDL-C (containing mainly triglyceride) and high LDL-C (containing mainly cholesterol) levels are therefore a recipe for forming, maintaining and enlarging plaques. They are justifiably called 'bad' lipids.

Where does HDL-C fit into this? The endothelium does try to heal itself and to get rid of the cholesterol and triglyceride gathering around it like a microscopic blackhead. The only way it can do that is to make the LDL-C and the VLDL-C even more dense. Only by collecting the fats into high-density lipoprotein masses – by turning VLDL-C and LDL-C into HDL-C – can the endothelium manage to extrude the fats from their deposits in the artery walls back into the bloodstream. Once in the bloodstream, the only organ to take it up in any serious amount is the liver, which can then turn it into bile and excrete it.

So, HDL-C is the body's answer to excessive fat deposits: it is made by the endothelium to protect itself. A high HDL-C means that there is a good turnover of lipids in the body, in the direction of lowering fatty deposits in the artery walls. HDL-C is justifiably the 'good' cholesterol.

In Summary

How can we bring all these facts about cholesterol and blood lipids together? The first message is that the higher your total cholesterol, the more likely you are to have a heart attack and/or stroke, and to have it earlier, rather than later, in your life. The second message is that TC is not the only risk. TC is only a rough guide. Within it are VLDL-C (mainly triglyceride), LDL-C (mainly cholesterol), and HDL-C. Raise the first two, and lower the third, and you make a heart attack and/or stroke more likely. Lower the first two and raise the third, and you reduce your chance of a heart attack and/or stroke.

Most of today's management of people with a high cholesterol or any of the other forms of dyslipidaemia, therefore, is devoted to the second aim – to lowerTG and LDL-C and, if possible, to raise HDL-C at the same time. How we do that is the whole point of this book. But, just in case you aren't convinced, the next chapter describes the evidence that has led us to these very definite goals.

ChapterThree

The Evidence for
Lowering Cholesterol

Medical textbooks on the relationship between blood lipid levels and heart disease and strokes run to thousands of pages, and refer to hundreds of huge studies done in different countries, races and cultures, and different social groups within countries. They review trials in which groups of healthy people who, untreated, are followed up until they die. They report trials of preventive management in healthy people who are at risk because of their dyslipidaemias (see Chapter Two), and of the treatment given people who are already getting symptoms suggestive of early heart disease or damage to the arteries of the brain.

One chapter of a book intended for non-medical readers could not possibly do justice to all these studies and trials, so I have picked instead a few of the studies that really made a difference to our understanding of lipids and how they affect health. This chapter gives the evidence on which today's management of high blood lipid levels is now based. It's a great detective story and I hope you find it as fascinating as I do.

The International Atherosclerosis Project

Like all good detective stories, it begins with a death. Or many millions of deaths, to be precise. In the 1950s, concern about the rising numbers of deaths from heart disease (they worried less about strokes then) led to the International Atherosclerosis Project. Between 1960 and 1965, researchers from 14 countries in the Americas, the Philippines, Jamaica, South Africa and Norway collected, at post-mortem, specimens of arteries from 22,509 people aged from 10 to 69 years who had died from diseases other than heart disease. They were all examined in one central laboratory.

The examinations showed that everyone – even the youngest – had some degree of atheroma, those yellow fatty streaks mentioned in Chapter One. Although the streaks were universal, the raised roughened plaques under the endothelium, thought to be the second stage of the disease, were not. They were much more common in certain communities, and when most severe (with many more plaques of larger size, often blocking arteries) were more common in particular geographic locations. What mattered was not race or gender, but the total amount of calories that had been eaten in food every day by the deceased. Remember, these specimens were not from people who had died from heart disease. Interestingly, the International Atherosclerosis Project did not find a link between obesity and the severity of the atheroma.

The authors concluded that almost everyone has some degree of atheroma, and that it develops slowly and quietly until it reaches a certain 'threshold' of severity. When the plaques are widespread enough and numerous enough to start to narrow important arteries in the heart and brain, only then does a person start to have symptoms, such as pain in the chest, or transient fainting attacks (signs of poor circulation in the brain).

They concluded that the disease was a mixture of inheritance and environment. Those most affected seemed to have inherited a pattern of lipids that helped promote atheroma, and this was complicated by overeating, which delivered an excess of fat to the arteries.

The Seven Countries Study

The Seven Countries Study was set up at around the same time by Professor Ancel Keys, of Minneapolis. He got together scientists from the United States, Japan, Finland, Italy, The Netherlands, Greece and Yugoslavia, who collected information on 12,763 men aged 40 to 59 between 1957 and 1962. They showed conclusively that total serum cholesterol (TC) (serum is blood plasma with the clotting materials removed) was the key to heart disease risk in every country. For example, in countries where blood pressures tended to be high, as long as the TC was low there was little heart disease. In countries where most men smoked (such as Japan), as long as the TC was low, again heart disease was uncommon. However, the combination of high blood pressure, smoking and a high TC multiplied the risks of heart disease several-fold.

The Finns stood out in this study. They indulged in much more physical activity than men in most of the other countries, a habit that before the study would have marked them out for a low heart attack rate. However, it did not protect them against heart disease – because their TCs were high.

The Seven Countries Study was the first definitely to link a high TC with the percentage of animal (saturated) fats in food. The Finns ate far more meat and dairy products than the other nationals: the consequence was a higher average TC and a much higher death rate from heart disease.

Saturated and Polyunsaturated Fats

Saturation is a chemical term relating to the number of hydrogen atoms in fat molecules. There are more in a saturated fat, fewer in a polyunsaturated fat. The chemistry does not need further explanation here, other than that the cholesterol made from saturated fats tends to be more easily deposited as plaque material. Cholesterol made from polyunsaturated fats and oils tends to be protective, like HDL-C. Saturated fats are in red meats and dairy products; polyunsaturated fats and oils are found in fish and vegetable oils. The low rate of heart disease in Japanese people was linked for the first time by the Seven Countries Study to their dependence on fish as their main source of fat.

These two international studies listed for the first time, too, the three main indicators of susceptibility – in any community – to heart disease:

1. Mean (average) serum TC level
2. The amount of atheroma in the coronary arteries
3. The ratio of polyunsaturated to saturated fats (the P/S ratio) in the diet.

A low P/S (of about 0.2, as in Finland – and Scotland) indicates food high in animal fats, and a high P/S ratio (of around 1, as in Japan) indicates food low in animal fats.

These three factors are closely linked. As the P/S ratio falls from 1 to 0.2, the serum TC rises, and so does the amount of atheroma in the arteries. As night follows day, so do the deaths from heart disease, particularly if you add smoking, uncontrolled high blood pressure and diabetes to the 'mix' of risks.

However, we cannot conclude that heart disease is just down to diet, and that if we all avoid animal fats we will avoid heart disease. In any case, few people brought up on an 'unhealthy', fatty diet would completely give up their burger and chips for a mackerel salad. Even when they do alter their eating habits in the right direction, it is rare for them to be able to bring down their TC levels by an amount that would substantially lower their risk of a heart attack.

The Framingham Heart Study

The Framingham Heart Study began in 1948 in the small town of Framingham, near Boston, Massachusetts. This study has become a byword in medical circles for excellence in its science and accuracy. It has followed more than 5,000 Framingham residents for their lifetimes. They are seen every two years until they die, and their cause of death is recorded. By the 1970s, the Framingham records had made it clear that a higher-than-average total cholesterol (TC) level in both men and women raised their risks of an early death due to heart disease. However, it was the first study to show how important the different forms of cholesterol are. After 16 years of follow-up of men who had entered the study at age 40, the researchers were able to create a profile of those who were at a high and low risk of developing coronary heart disease within the next six years.

The low-risk subjects were the non-smokers who had no sign of early diabetes and had no changes on their electrocardiogram suggestive of impending heart disease even when they had high blood pressure. Those at high risk were smokers, those who did not handle glucose well (so might be heading for diabetes), and those who showed some heart muscle thickening with their high blood pressure. Framingham also showed that the strong relationship between total cholesterol (TC) level and heart disease was even stronger for LDL-C: high LDL-C levels were an even better predictor of impending heart attack than a high TC.

The British Regional Heart Study

In Britain the most impressive work in the field of heart disease and cholesterol has been the British Regional Heart Study, the main instigator, overseer and author of which is Professor A. G. Shaper, of the Royal Free Hospital, the University of London. It has followed 7,735 men aged 40 to 59, from the late 1970s until now. They are drawn from 24 towns in the main regions of England, Scotland and Wales. Professor Shaper and his colleagues divided the men into five groups according to their TC levels, dividing the TC measurements into equal fifths. They calculated from their findings that, in the first five years of follow-up, the men in the top fifth of the range of cholesterol levels would have 59 per cent of the heart attacks suffered by the entire group. Only 7 per cent of the heart attacks would occur in the men in the lowest two-fifths of the TC range. Bringing cholesterol levels down from high levels should, it was thought, greatly lower this risk. However, as there are many more men in the middle fifths than in the highest fifth, any strategy to lower overall heart attacks must be designed to lower cholesterol levels even in them. Professor Shaper is a strong advocate of making the whole population aware that they should try to lower their own cholesterol levels.

Other Studies

Many other studies have come to the same conclusion. The Multiple Risk Factor Intervention Trial, ingeniously called MRFIT, showed that the risk of heart attack rises over the whole range of TC levels, from the lowest to the highest. It added that the biggest component in that risk is LDL-C. Five large trials (under the titles of WOSCOPS, 4S, CARE, PLAC-1 and REGRESS) have reported that reducing the LDL-C with a statin drug lowers the heart attack rate by between 24 and 37 per cent compared with treatment with a placebo. These findings were so significant that it would now be impossible to use a placebo in any trial of cholesterol-lowering drugs. (For more about these trials, see Chapter Seven.)

It has been more difficult to prove a close relationship between changes in HDL-C or triglyceride (TG) and heart disease. TG levels tend to go in the opposite direction to HDL-C, so it is difficult to prove that one of them alone is responsible for disease. Measuring TG is also a problem, because levels can rise steeply soon after meals, and give a falsely high reading. So it is usual to measure them after an overnight fast.

Nevertheless, the Swedes have linked high plasma TG levels to a definitely raised risk of sudden death from heart attack in the Stockholm Prospective Study, as over the course of the study some 321 men and 55 women died – easily enough to prove their case. The higher their TG, after taking their HDL-C and LDL-C into account, the more at risk they were. That study, and another study from Framingham highlighted the fact that for women, perhaps TG was even more important than LDL-C in determining whether or not they developed heart disease.

By 1996, Drs J E Hokansen and M A Austin had brought together enough evidence from trials in which 46,000 men and 11,000 women had been followed for many years to confirm that higher plasma TG levels do pose a strong risk of heart disease. This risk, they showed, was quite independent of the HDL-C level. In fact, the Copenhagen Male Study, which followed 2,900 men for eight years, 229 of whom had first heart attacks during the study, showed that, contrary to its protective effects in people with high LDL-C levels, HDL-C did not protect against heart attacks linked to a high TG.

Why should a high TG level be so lethal? It is linked to a poorer-than-normal ability to control blood glucose levels properly – in fact a 'pre-diabetic' state, in which there may also be high blood pressure and high levels of insulin in the blood.

Happily, today's treatment to lower TG and LDL-C levels does work. It not only does the job of lowering blood levels of these two 'bad' lipids, but in doing so it also definitely reduces the numbers of heart attacks and strokes. We showed this in my home area, in the West of Scotland Coronary Prevention Study (WOSCOPS). Men with TG levels above 1.6 mmol/l benefited more from the drug treatment (in WOSCOPS it was a statin) than did those with TC levels above 7 mmol/l, although both groups on the treatment had substantially fewer heart attacks and strokes than those given a placebo.

Possibly the most surprising result of all was in the Stockholm Ischaemic Heart Disease Secondary Prevention Study, in which patients three months after a heart attack were given lipid-lowering treatment or followed as 'controls' for five years. The death rate among those given the treatment was 26 per cent lower than that among the controls. However, there were 60 per cent fewer deaths from heart attacks among those whose TG levels were lowered by more than 30 per cent by the treatment.

So it is abundantly clear that if you have a higher-than-normal LDL-C or TG, and a lower-than-normal HDL-C, you should correct these abnormalities if you wish to avoid a heart attack or stroke. How to go about this is described in Chapter Ten. The next chapter, however, is about you, personally. It describes how doctors detect dyslipidaemias, and how people with them are investigated. It is no longer just a matter of measuring TC and putting people on a 'diet', and then waiting to see if it works. That time has gone. There are guidelines for every general practitioner to follow, and they are described next.

Chapter Four

Making the Diagnosis

The big problem for doctors in diagnosing cases of hyperlipidaemia is that most people with it have no symptoms and do not know that they are virtually sitting on a time bomb. So the vast majority of people who are being treated for their high total cholesterol (TC), high low-density lipoprotein cholesterol (LDL-C) or high triglyceride (TG) were only found to have these problems after a routine blood test, as might be done at a 'well-man' or 'well-woman' clinic for people over 40, or for an insurance medical, or when investigating another illness.

In the past, screening for blood cholesterol used to be done when people reached middle age, some time between their 40th and 50th birthdays. That was a haphazard approach, and led to many early cases of hyperlipidaemia being missed. The guidelines for screening today for cholesterol by general practitioners in Britain are clearly set out by the Royal College of General Practitioners (RCGP). The RCGP has set priority groups for cholesterol screening as follows:

Group 1

People under 65 already known to have symptoms of heart disease or peripheral vascular disease (circulation disorders in the limbs)

People with the clinical signs of hypercholesterolaemia (these are described below)

People with relatives who have or had cholesterol problems, or had early heart attacks or other diseases linked to atheroma (like early strokes or circulation problems)

People with diseases linked to abnormal cholesterol levels, such as diabetes, thyroid failure and kidney disease.

Group 2 People known to show at least two of the following risks for heart disease: smoking, high blood pressure, obesity and male gender

Group 3 Those with a single risk factor from the list in group 2

Group 4 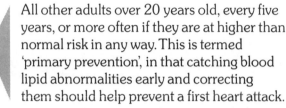 All other adults over 20 years old, every five years, or more often if they are at higher than normal risk in any way. This is termed 'primary prevention', in that catching blood lipid abnormalities early and correcting them should help prevent a first heart attack.

People in the first two priority groups should be offered the works – a full fasting lipid profile (that is, detailed blood lipid analysis of a sample taken 12 hours after the last meal). This profile should measure TC, HDL-C and LDL-C and TG.

Taking the blood sample is, of course, just a small part of the screening consultation. You must be prepared to answer several questions about your family. They include:

Your parents' ages, or age at death, their lipid profile (if they/ you know it) and whether they have, or had, a disease caused by atheroma
Information about cholesterol-linked illnesses in other close relatives, like grandparents, uncles and aunts, or siblings
The illnesses close relatives have died from
Of those who died from atheroma-linked diseases, other risk factors, such as: did they smoke or have high blood pressure or diabetes?

Next comes the examination. A few people do show skin problems that signal that they have hyperlipidaemia. Recently I met an old friend for the first time in 10 years. I noticed that he had little raised fatty streaks on both upper eyelids, near the margin with the nose. He admitted that they had appeared within the previous two years. As he was now 55, he thought they were just a part of the ageing process.

He was wrong. They were small 'xanthomas', or, more accurately because they were on the eyelid, 'xanthelasmas'. These are fatty deposits in the skin due to a raised cholesterol level. He was slim and was dubious about seeing his doctor about such a small thing. However, my worries were justified when he found that his TC was over 9.5mmol/l, giving him a very high risk of a heart attack in the next few years. He is now on a statin drug, with a TC below 4.5mmol/l, and his heart attack risk is a tenth of what it was.

My friend is one of the people who have inherited their abnormal blood lipid levels. They have *primary hyperlipidaemia* and they are usually diagnosed at a younger age than my friend, because they show some signs that are pointers to the disease, even in childhood in some cases, and they become ill earlier.

The Primary Hyperlipidaemias

The primary, or familial (because they run in families) hyperlipidae-mias are classified according to which particular aspect of the lipid profile is abnormal. So there are people with familial hypercholester-olaemia, with familial defective apolipoprotein B, with 'type III' hyperlipoproteinaemia, and with hypertriglyceridaemia. Doctors skilled in their diagnosis may spot them in the surgery waiting room, because they may show very specific signs of their problem.

Familial Hypercholesterolaemia (FH)
Much depends on whether the gene for FH has been inherited from one parent (this is called heterozygous inheritance) or from both (homozygous). Homozygotes (people who carry the FH gene from both parents) are usually spotted in childhood, because they grow xanthomas (raised fatty lumps in the skin) in the webs between the fingers, behind the knees or on the outer aspects of the knees or elbows.

Heterozygotes for FH don't start to have symptoms and signs of their disease until at least teenage or their early twenties. An early sign is recurrent inflammation (swelling and tenderness) of the Achilles tendon, usually with exercise. Later FH heterozygotes grow xanthomas on the tendons, and they can appear, too, on the tendons of the hands, below the kneecaps and around the elbow. If you find you can't get shoes that fit because of lumps on your feet, get your cholesterol level checked. This is a fairly common first sign of familial FH.

About one in five people with familial FH grow xanthelasmas, like my friend, on their eyelids. They may also show a white rim around their iris before they are 35. This white rim is called 'arcus senilis' (the arc of old age) because it is very common in old age. Anyone with such a white rim at a young age should have their lipid levels checked.

If you are growing xanthomas or xanthelasmas, don't opt for surgery unless you really have to. If you correct your blood lipid profile, they will subside and eventually disappear, mostly within a year and often within six months. Happily nowadays it is usually easy to do just that.

Familial Defective Apolipoprotein B
People with this fault in their lipid profile have hypercholesterolaemia which follows a similar pattern to that of familial FH. They often produce an arcus senilis when quite young (even in their teens) and they tend to grow xanthomas and xanthelasmas.

Type III Hyperlipoproteinaemia
This is a rare form of dyslipidaemia, making up only 1 per cent of all inherited lipid disorders, in which there is an increase in 'intermediate density' lipoproteins (or IDL) in the blood. They have high TC and TG levels. People with it usually see their doctors because they start to grow grape-like bunches of solid fatty lumps on the outer skin of the elbows. As these grow bigger, they join together into a larger lump. These are called 'tuberous' xanthomas, in an unflattering comparison with potatoes. The diagnosis is supported by a yellow or even orange staining in the creases in the palms of the hands.

Primary Hypertriglyceridaemia
People with this form of dyslipidaemia can show astonishingly high TG levels without having any outward sign or suffering any symptoms from it. Normally, TG levels are under 2mmol/l: it is only when they rise above 20mmol/l that people start to feel ill with it. Then they may feel tenderness in the upper abdomen, under the rib margins, as the liver (on the right) and the spleen (on the left), swell with the extra load of fat. When the TG rises above 40mmol/l, a rash

of small raised white or yellow spots may appear over the buttocks, arms and thighs.

Measuring Lipids – At What Level Are They Abnormal?

So, you are suspected of having a dyslipidaemia, and your blood is tested. As yet you have no problems and look upon yourself as healthy. What levels of the different lipids are accepted as normal and when do you need to worry? Probably the best way to illustrate this is with a table. However, the table is not appropriate for people who already know they have heart disease or diabetes. They should keep their LDL-C under 2.6mmol/l, and keep their LDL-C to HDL-C ratio under 2.5. If it is over 3, it is too high. Regardless of whether or not you already have symptoms of heart disease, you should try to keep your TC to HDL-C ratio below 3.5. It is too high if it is above 4.

Lipid levels outside the normal range are more dangerous (pose more of a risk) if you are young, have diabetes, smoke, have high blood pressure, have an 'apple' type obesity, or have relatives who have died early from heart disease. So if have one of these extra risk factors, and you know your lipid levels are sticking in the 'raised' or 'very high' categories, please do your utmost to reduce them.

Table: Levels of lipids (mmol/l) in people with no known heart disease

	Normal	On the edge (needs watching)	Raised (needs treating)	Very high (needs urgent attention)
TC	under 5	5 to 6.2	6.3 to 7.8	more than 7.8
LDL-C	under 3	3 to 4.1	4.2 to 5.5	more than 5.5
TG –				
(men)	under 2	2 to 2.5	2.5 to 11	more than 11
(women)	under 1.5	1.5 to 2	2 to 11	more than 11
HDL-C –				
(men)	over 1.1	below 1.1		
(women)	over 1.3	below 1.3		

(To convert to North American units of mg/dl, multiply cholesterol by 40 and TG by 90.)

There is an official classification of hyperlipidaemias, called the Fredrickson system, which was developed at the US National Institutes of Health. You may notice the diagnosis on your blood test form. Its complexity is outside the scope of this book; it is enough to state that it classes people according to raised levels of different lipoproteins, triglyceride and cholesterol, and on how greatly they are raised.

Fredrickson Type 2b, in which LDL, VLDL, TG and cholesterol are all raised, accounts for 40 per cent of all patients with hyperlipidaemia. Type 4, in which VLDL, but not LDL, is raised, along with high TG and cholesterol levels, occurs in 45 per cent. Ten per cent have type 2a hyperlipidaemia, in which LDL and cholesterol, but not VLDL or TG, are raised. Type 4 hyperlipidaemia is less 'atherogenic' (leading to less endothelial damage, and therefore less likely to cause heart attacks) than either form of Type 2. Type 3, mentioned above with its grape-like xanthomas and yellow skin palm creases, in which high IDL is the problem, is very atherogenic, so that untreated it leads to early heart disease, but it accounts for fewer than 1 per cent of all cases of hyperlipidaemia. Types 1 and 5 hyperlipidaemia are very rare, and are not very atherogenic, even though the TG level in type 5, in which VLDL is raised, can be very high.

Secondary Hyperlipidaemias – Finding the Cause

Once you have the news that your blood lipids are not what they should be, it is not simply a question of starting treatment to lower them. Most hyperlipidaemias are not primary (i.e. not inherited) but secondary (arising out of the complications of another disease). So your doctor will want to perform tests to rule out these other diseases, of which there are quite a few, among them diabetes, kidney disease, liver and gall-bladder disease, thyroid disease (usually an underactive thyroid), and less common diseases such as Cushing's syndrome (overactivity of part of the adrenal gland, causing overproduction of cortisone) and intermittent porphyria. So you will be asked to give more blood, to check for all these.

One common cause of high levels of combined cholesterol and triglyceride (in which the TG level can be five times the upper limit of normal) is drugs prescribed for other conditions. For example, oestrogens given in the contraceptive pill or as hormone replacement in and after the menopause can cause this pattern of hyperlipidaemia. So can thiazide diuretics and beta-blocker drugs given for high blood pressure, and cortisone-like drugs given, say, for allergies, for various chronic illnesses, and after transplant surgery.

One other cause of this type of combined hyperlipidaemia is over-indulgence in alcohol. Your doctor will confirm this by measuring your blood levels of substances called *transferases*, which give a close estimate of how much you have been drinking daily over the previous three to six months. You can't cheat on the test by stopping drinking the night before! If you have high liver transferase levels and your liver shows other damage due to alcohol, then an important part of your life from now on is to avoid it.

If one of these reasons for your hyperlipidaemia turns up in your test results, then the first principle in medical treatment is to treat the cause. Your doctor will take the appropriate action for each primary cause, and in many cases the cholesterol or triglyceride problem will take care of itself. You will probably have to keep checking on it, with regular blood tests, for the rest of your life.

However, it must be said that by far the most common cause of secondary hyperlipidaemia is over-eating. If you eat a lot of fatty foods, then you will fill your bloodstream with fat, and that, in turn, has to settle somewhere. It will either be stored in your already over-burdened fat storage cells around your middle and on your back, bottom and hips, or it will be deposited in your artery walls. You do not have to be born with the tendency to atheroma to develop it. If you eat more than you can expend in energy output, you will put on fat. So for the vast majority of people with dyslipidaemia, the cause is easy to find. The cure, however, is much more difficult.

Chapter Five

Putting Things Right –
A Complete Approach

The constant theme throughout this book is that you cannot treat your high cholesterol levels in isolation. It is no use just popping a cholesterol-lowering pill and carrying on with your life as it was before. You must take stock of everything you do and, where your lifestyle is putting you at risk, change it.

Above all else, for most people the way to improve cholesterol levels is to adopt healthy eating habits. I have studiously avoided the word 'diet' here, because it is notoriously impossible to stick to one. This has to be a true change in your living habits that can't be described as a diet, but a new way of life, as if you have emigrated to another country and have had to adapt to the lifestyle of your new nation.

And the lifestyle changes you need to make are not, in any case, just about what you eat. They are also about weight control, stopping smoking, drinking less alcohol and increasing exercise. If you are not at a high immediate risk of a heart attack, and after adopting all these lifestyle changes you have not within three months substantially reduced your blood lipid levels, then you will be offered lipid-lowering drugs. Of course, if your doctor believes your blood lipid problem is putting you at high risk, then you will be offered drug treatment much sooner. But the drug treatment is not an alternative to the new lifestyle: it is to be taken along with it.

The rule of thumb is to give drugs immediately to those with severe primary (familial – see the last chapter) hypercholesterolaemia, because changing their eating habits makes very little difference to their lipid levels. Drugs (usually a fibrate – see Chapter Seven) are also given to people found to have very high fasting TG levels (usually above 10mmol/l). Drugs are also given immediately to people with hyperlipidaemia who already have had heart symptoms such as angina, or a heart attack. This is particularly important for people with early heart disease who have been found to have familial dyslipidaemias: usually the drugs are started after first measuring their fasting LDL-C levels on two separate occasions.

Eating Healthily

If you have a high blood lipid profile, regardless of whether you have a high total cholesterol, triglyceride, LDL-C or VLDL-C, the management of your eating habits should be the same. Most general practices now have a dietician attached to them, so that you can get the fine details of how to go about changing your eating with her (I wonder why there are so few male dieticians?). This section of the book deals therefore with the general principles, rather than the details.

The first principle is that the new way of eating must be enjoyable and sustainable. Otherwise you will backslide into your old habits very quickly. So make sure that you find a new eating lifestyle that you enjoy and will keep on enjoying. Now read carefully through the next few paragraphs. They list the elements of eating that are important for you to understand as principles. Only after understanding *why* you have to make changes can you truly succeed in doing so.

The Principles of Your New Eating Habits

Your Total Fat Intake
If you replace a substantial amount of the fat you used to eat with foods made up largely of complex carbohydrates (like starches and complex sugars – as in bread, potatoes, pasta, rice and green and root vegetables) you will help yourself to lose any obesity and reduce your intake of saturated fats. All fats, remember, whether saturated or polyunsaturated, give you the same amount of calories per gram.
Saturated Fats
The more saturated fat you eat, the higher will be your blood cholesterol, your LDL-C and your risk of a heart attack.

The P/S Ratio
Monounsaturated and polyunsaturated fats are just as rich in calories as saturated fats, but they lower cholesterol levels when you switch to them from saturated fats. Monounsaturated fats, as in olive oil, help to raise HDL-C levels more than do polyunsaturated fats (and are

therefore probably more beneficial). This may help to explain why heart attacks are rare in countries around the Mediterranean.

Cholesterol-rich Foods
Eating a lot of cholesterol-rich foods, such as eggs and liver, can raise your blood cholesterol level, particularly when you also eat a lot of saturated fats. However, people differ widely in their response to cholesterol in their food. For some the amount eaten makes little difference to their blood levels, in others it causes a steep rise. As we make enough cholesterol in our livers to do us, there is no need to eat cholesterol-rich food.

Overweight
If you have stored too much body fat – that is, you are overweight – then you will be prone to high blood pressure, high cholesterol and TG levels, and 'insulin resistance', which is a state, if it continues, that will lead to diabetes. If you are fat to the extent you are more than 10 per cent overweight for your height, then you are already at a heightened risk, even if you are a young adult, of coronary disease.

Exercise
Increase your amount of regular physical activity, and you will help control your weight, in the meantime increasing your HDL-C levels – which you know by now, of course, to be beneficial and to protect against heart disease. The recommendation by all the experts is to do aerobic exercise (walking, running, cycling, swimming, dancing) for 20 minutes or more, four to five times a week.

Alcohol
Alcohol in moderate amounts may raise HDL-C levels, which is beneficial, but it also raises TG levels, which is not! So drink any alcohol in moderation. Excess alcohol (more than 2-3 drinks a day, more than 4-5 days a week, or binge-drinking at weekends) is damaging, and not beneficial to the heart or endothelium. Most of the publicity about alcohol recently is that red wine is good for the heart. The problem is that the amount that is actually good for you is much smaller than many people drink in an evening. Remember that the usual drink poured out in a private house is much more than the standard drink poured in a hotel, restaurant or pub.

So how do you put your principles into practice? Here is a list of goals to help you to do so.

1. Reduce your fat intake to no more than 30 per cent of your total calorie intake in the day. Divide the fats equally into polyunsaturated, monounsaturated and saturated, so that each component takes up 10 per cent of your calorie intake.
2. Increase your dietary fibre intake, so that you eat more pulses, other vegetables and fruit.
3. Reduce your intake of foods rich in cholesterol so that you are not eating more than 300mg per day.
4. Increase your intake of complex carbohydrates (bread, cereals, fruit, vegetables) to make up 55 per cent of your calorie intake.
5. Take salt only in very moderate amounts. Don't have a salt cellar on the table, and don't add much to your cooking. This should lower your blood pressure.
6. Restrict alcohol to 2 to 3 small drinks a day, preferably on only 4 to 5 days a week at most. Never binge-drink.
7. If you are overweight, reduce it using the above principles and more exercise.

This advice is difficult to follow. After all, how many of us would know what 10 per cent of our calorie intake is, or how many eggs (or other foods) provide 300mg of cholesterol? And measuring and weighing food takes the pleasure out of preparing and eating it. As you must retain pleasure in your eating, here are some tips to make things easier for you.

Choosing Your Food

Dairy Products
Use skimmed or semi-skimmed milk and other low-fat products. Use yoghurt instead of cream, and soft margarine labelled 'high in' monounsaturates and/or polyunsaturates, rather than butter. Cook in vegetable oil labelled in the same way. Use cottage curd cheeses rather than cream cheeses or hard cheeses such as cheddar, which are high in fat.

Meat
Grill or bake lean meat, rather than frying it. Eat poultry, but first remove the skin, which is high in fat. Avoid prepared meats such as sausages and pâtès.

Fish
Replace meat on around three days a week with fish, especially oily fish such as herring, sardines, mackerel, tuna, salmon and trout. Fish oils improve the lipid profile in subtle ways, and many trials have shown that people who eat a lot of oily fish have substantially fewer heart attacks than those who mostly eat meat.

Eggs
Eat no more than three egg yolks per week, including eggs used in prepared foods. Egg whites are cholesterol-free, so consider using them and an egg substitute in cooking instead.

Bread, Cakes and Cereals
Use wholemeal or high-fibre, rather than white bread. Eat wholemeal (or wholewheat – the two words seem now to be interchangeable) breakfast cereals, pasta and brown rice. Do not buy cakes (they are full of sugar and fat) and use wholemeal flour, with less sugar and fat, when baking for yourself.

Fruit and Vegetables
You can indulge in as many vegetables and fruits as you like, provided you don't eat so many that you become overweight.

Foods high in total fat	All fried foods, regardless of the type of oil or fat in which they have been fried. Whole milk, cream, high-fat cheeses and fatty red meats, particularly manufactured sausages, meat pies and pâtés.
Foods high in cholesterol	Liver, offal, egg yolks.
Foods high in saturated fat	Fatty meats and their products, as above. Foods cooked in butter, hard margarines, lard, suet or dripping. Coconut and palm oils.

47

Foods high in polyunsaturated fats (better for you than saturated fats)	Most nuts and seeds, oily fish such as sardines, pilchards, herring, mackerel, tuna, trout and salmon. Most vegetable oils and soft margarines.
Foods high in monounsaturated fat	Olives and olive oil.

Chapter Six

WhyYou Mustn't Smoke – and How to Stop IfYou Do

I have mentioned the bad effects of smoking earlier in this book. If you have hyperlipidaemia of any type, you are mad to smoke, because it makes your health much worse and brings closer the day you succumb to heart disease. So if you are a smoker, this is the most important chapter in the book for you. You must be a non-smoker before you put this book down.

Smoking is a stupid, suicidal habit for anyone, no matter how healthy. It is even worse, if that is possible, for people with hyperlipidaemia of any kind, because it multiplies all the extra risks they face of heart disease, strokes and kidney disease.

How Smoking Harms You

Tobacco smoke contains carbon monoxide and nicotine. The first poisons the red blood cells, so that they cannot pick up and distribute much-needed oxygen to the organs and tissues, including the heart muscle. Carbon monoxide-affected red cells (in the 20-a-day smoker, nearly 20 per cent of red cells are carrying carbon monoxide instead of oxygen) are also stiffer than normal, so that they can't bend and flex through the smallest blood vessels. The gas also directly poisons the heart muscle, so that it cannot contract properly and efficiently, thereby delivering a 'double whammy' of damage which a hyperlipidaemic heart – already possibly working under the disadvantage of multiple plaques of atheroma in the coronary arteries – can ill afford.

Nicotine causes small arteries to narrow, so that the blood flow through them slows. It raises blood cholesterol levels, thickening the blood and promoting the degenerative process in the endothelium of the small arteries – a process which is already faster than normal in people with hyperlipidaemia.

Both nicotine and carbon monoxide encourage the blood to clot, multiplying the risks of coronary thrombosis and a thrombotic stroke even more.

Add to all this the tars that smoke deposits in the lungs, which further reduce the ability of red cells to pick up oxygen, and the scars and damage to the endothelium in the lungs that always lead to chronic bronchitis – and often to cancer – and you have a formula for disaster.

The Bald Facts

If these facts about smoking do not convince you to stop, then you may as well give up reading this book, because there is no point in being 'health conscious' if you continue to indulge in tobacco. Its ill-effects will counterbalance any good that your doctors can do for you.

- Smoking causes more deaths from heart attacks than from lung cancer or bronchitis.
- People who smoke have two or three times the risk of a fatal heart attack than non-smokers. The risk rises with the numbers of cigarettes smoked, and is multiplied many times over if you also have hyperlipidaemia.
- Men under 45 who smoke 25 or more cigarettes a day have a 10- to 15-times greater chance of death from a heart attack than non-smoking men of the same age.
- About 40 per cent of all heavy smokers die before they reach 65. Of those who reach that age, many are disabled by bronchitis, angina, heart failure and leg amputations, all because they smoked. A high cholesterol and/or triglyceride level makes all these risks of smoking much greater. Only 10 per cent of smokers survive in reasonable health to the age of 75. Most non-smokers reach 75 in good health.
- In Britain, 40 per cent of all cancer deaths are from lung cancer, which is very rare in non-smokers. Of 441 British male doctors who died from lung cancer, only seven had never smoked. Only one non-smoker in 60 develops lung cancer: The figure for heavy smokers is one in six!
- Other cancers more common in smokers than in non-smokers include tongue, throat, larynx, pancreatic, kidney, bladder and cervical cancers.

The very fact that you are reading this book means that you are taking an intelligent interest in your health. So after reading so far, it should be common sense to you not to smoke. Yet it is very difficult to stop, and many people who need an excuse for not stopping put up various arguments for their stance. Here are ones that every doctor is tired of hearing, and my replies:

My father/grandfather smoked 20 a day and lived till he was 75.

Everyone knows someone like that, but they conveniently forget the many others they have known who died long before their time. The chances are that you will be one of them, rather than one of the lucky few.

People who don't smoke also have heart attacks.

True. There are other causes of heart attacks, but 70 per cent of all people under 65 admitted to coronary care with heart attacks are smokers, as are 91 per cent of people with angina considered for coronary bypass surgery.

I believe in moderation in all things, and I only smoke moderately.

That's rubbish. We don't accept moderation in mugging, or dangerous driving, or exposure to asbestos (which, incidentally, causes far fewer deaths from lung cancer than smoking). Younger men who are only moderate smokers have a much higher risk of heart attack than non-smoking men of the same age.

I can cut down on cigarettes, but I can't stop.

It won't do you much good if you do. People who cut down usually inhale more from each cigarette and leave a smaller butt, so that they end up with the same blood levels of nicotine and carbon monoxide. You must stop completely.

I'm just as likely to be run over in the road as to die from my smoking.

In Britain about 15 people die on the roads each day. This contrasts with 100 deaths a day from lung cancer, 100 from chronic bronchitis and 100 from heart attacks, almost all of which are due to smoking. Of every 1,000 young men who smoke, on average one will be murdered, six will die on the roads, and 250 will die from their smoking habit. Increase those risks for men and women with diabetes who also smoke.

I have to die from something.
In my experience this is always said by someone in good health. They no longer say it after their heart attack or stroke, or after they have coughed up blood.

I don't want to be old, anyway.
We define 'old' differently as we grow older. Most of us would like to live a long time, without the inconvenience of being old. If we take care of ourselves on the way to becoming old, we have at least laid the foundations for enjoying our old age.

I'd rather die of a heart attack than something else.
Most of us would like a fast, sudden death, but many heart attack victims leave a grieving partner in their early 50s to face 30 years of loneliness. Is that really what you wish?

Stress, not smoking, is the main cause of heart attacks.
Not true. Stress is very difficult to measure and it is very difficult to relate to heart attack rates. In any case, you have to cope with stress, whether you smoke or not. Smoking is an extra burden that can never help, and it does not relieve stress. It isn't burning the candle at both ends that causes harm, but burning the cigarette at one end.

I'll stop when I start to feel ill.
That would be fine if the first sign of illness were not a full-blown heart attack from which more than a third die in the first 4 hours. It's too late to stop then.

I'll put on weight if I stop smoking.
You probably will, because your appetite will return and you will be able to taste food again. But if you have read the section in this book about changing your eating habits to control your lipid levels, then you will lose any extra weight anyway. In any case, the benefits of stopping smoking far outweigh the few extra pounds you may put on.

I enjoy smoking and don't want to give it up.
Is that really true? Is that not just an excuse because you can't stop? Ask yourself what your real pleasure is in smoking, and try to be honest with the answer.

Cigarettes settle my nerves. If I stopped I'd have to take a tranquilliser.
Smoking is a prop, like a baby's dummy, but it solves nothing. It doesn't remove any causes of stress, and only makes things worse because it adds a promoter of bad health. And when you start to have symptoms, like the regular morning cough, it only makes you worry more.

I'll change to a pipe or cigar – they are safer.
Lifelong pipe and cigar smokers are less prone than cigarette smokers to heart attacks, but have five times the risk of lung cancer and ten times the risk of chronic bronchitis than non-smokers. Cigarette smokers who switch to pipes or cigars continue to be at high risk of heart attack, probably because they inhale.

I've been smoking for 30 years – it's too late to stop now.
It's not too late, whenever you stop. The risk of sudden death from a first heart attack falls away very quickly after stopping, even after a lifetime of smoking. If you stop after surviving a heart attack then you halve the risk of a second. It takes longer to reduce your risk of lung cancer, but it falls by 80 per cent over the next 15 years, no matter how long you have been a smoker.

I wish I could stop. I've tried everything, but nothing has worked.
Stopping smoking isn't easy unless you really want to do it. You have to make the effort yourself, rather than think that someone else can do it for you. So you must be motivated. If the next few pages do not motivate you, then nothing will.

How to Stop Smoking

You must find the right reason for yourself to stop. For someone with hyperlipidaemia, one reason is that it will further reduce your high chance of having a heart attack. But there are plenty of other reasons.

If you are a teenager or in your early twenties, who sees middle-age and sickness as remote possibilities, and smoking as exciting and dangerous, the best way to stop is to think on the way it makes you look and smell. You can also add the environmental pollution of cigarette ends and the way big business exploits Third World nations, keeping their populations in poverty while they make huge profits by putting land that should be growing food under tobacco cultivation. Pakistan uses 120,000 acres, and Brazil half a million acres of their richest agricultural land to grow tobacco. As the multinationals are now promoting their product very heavily to the developing world, no young adult who smokes can claim to be really concerned about the health of the Third World. This may be more likely to persuade you to stop (or not to start) than any thought about health or looks.

Smoking ages people prematurely, causing wrinkles and giving a pale, pasty complexion. Women smokers experience the menopause at an earlier age, even in the mid-thirties, which can destroy the plans of businesswomen to have their families after a shot at a career. Smoking plus a high triglyceride level – an extremely common combination in women – vastly increases your chances of having a heart attack or stroke. It removes all your natural advantages over men in your protection against heart attack.

The statistics for non-hyperlipidaemic men and women in their 60s who smoke are frightening enough, without bringing in the extra burden of a high cholesterol or triglyceride level to further worsen them. More than a third of smoking men fail to reach pensionable age – add many more to that figure if they also have any form of hyperlipidaemia.

Let us assume you are now fully motivated. How do you stop? It is easy. You become a non-smoker, as if you have never smoked. You throw away all your cigarettes and decide never to buy or accept another one. Announce the fact to all your friends, who will usually support you, and that's that. Most people find that they don't have true withdrawal symptoms, provided they are happy to stop. A few become agitated, irritable, nervous and can't sleep at night. But people who have had to stop for medical reasons – say because they have been admitted to coronary care – hardly ever have withdrawal symptoms.

This strongly suggests that withdrawal symptoms are psychological, rather than physical. And if you are stopping because you have found you have a problem with your blood lipids, that is not too different from the coronary care scenario. If you can last a week or two without a smoke, you will probably never light up again. The desire to smoke will disappear as the levels of carbon monoxide, nicotine and tarry chemicals in your lungs, blood, brain and other organs gradually subside.

If you must stop gradually, plan ahead. Write down a diary of the cigarettes you will have, leaving out one or two each succeeding day, and stick to it. Carry nicotine chewing gum or get a patch if you must, but remember that the nicotine is still harmful. Don't look on it as a long-term alternative to a smoke. If you are having real difficulty stopping, ask your doctor for a prescription of Zyban. You may be offered a two-month course of the drug. It helps, but is by no means infallible.

If you do use aids to stop (others include acupuncture and hypnosis), remember they have no magical properties. They are a crutch to lean on while you make the determined effort to stop altogether. They cannot help if your will to stop is weak.

Recognise, too, that stopping smoking is not an end in itself. It is only part of your new way of life, which includes your new way of eating and exercise, and your new attitude to your future health. And you owe it not only to yourself but also to your partner, family and friends, because it will help to give them a healthier you, hopefully for years to come.

You are not on your own. More than a million Britons have stopped smoking each year for the last 15 years. Only one in three adults now smokes. By stopping , you are joining the sensible majority.

Chapter Seven

Drug Treatments

The next few chapters of this book are devoted to the use of prescription drugs to lower raised blood lipid levels. If you have hyperlipidaemia, you are probably already on one of these drugs, and you perhaps wonder whether they are doing more harm than good. This is a common problem for people who have few, if any, symptoms of disease, yet who are told they must take drugs for the rest of their life if they are to avoid future illness. They naturally fear that taking a drug, especially a new type of drug, for years may have unexpected damaging side-effects. Would it be worth stopping the drug and taking the chance that they won't get the predicted heart attack or stroke?

This chapter first sets out the recommendations by the European Joint Task Force (a group of distinguished specialists in lipid disorders) on who should be given lipid-lowering drugs. It then gives the evidence from trials which helped the Task Force come to its decisions, and leaves you to decide whether the benefits of the drugs outweigh the potential drawbacks. I must state here that if I had a dyslipidaemia I would certainly take the appropriate drug every day for the foreseeable future.

Who Should and Should Not Be Offered Drug Treatment

Unless you already have been ill with, or are showing early symptoms of, heart disease, if you have mild or moderate hypercholesterolaemia which has started to reverse after changing your lifestyle, you do not need drugs.

Nor do you need drugs to lower your lipid levels if you have hypertriglyceridaemia caused by another treatable condition. What you need is specific treatment for that illness.

According to the European Joint Task Force, you do need drug treatment if you:
are a high-risk patient, i.e. someone who already has shown
signs of heart disease.

have hypertriglyceridaemia with other risk factors such as high blood pressure.

are at high risk due to special risk factors, such as having high lipoprotein(a) or high fibrinogen levels in your blood. They both indicate fairly severe risk to your endothelium.

have hypercholesterolaemia that has not responded to changes in lifestyle designed to lower your cholesterol.

have severe hypertriglyceridaemia and pancreatitis, or are at risk of repeated attacks of pancreatitis. Pancreatitis is a serious inflammation of the pancreas, which lies in the upper abdomen and is involved in digesting proteins and producing insulin. Pancreatitis is common in hypertriglyceridaemia and, if unchecked, can lead to diabetes and severe digestive problems. It can be fatal.

have familial hyperlipidaemia, as it is unlikely to respond to lifestyle changes and carries a high risk of heart attack and stroke.

have any severe form of dyslipidaemia, or evidence of coronary disease along with mild or moderate dyslipidaemia.

You will gather from these guidelines that almost everyone with a lipid disorder is eligible for drug treatment. This must mean that the Task Force is convinced by the results of trials that drugs provide much more benefit than harm. Here is some of the evidence on which they've based that judgement.

The Air Force/Texas Coronary Atherosclerosis Prevention Study (AFCAPS/TexCAPS)

This study was reported to the American Heart Association in 1997. It followed 6,605 men and women with no initial evidence of heart disease. The women made up 15 per cent of the trial subjects.

At the start of the trial, both the men and women had low-density lipoprotein cholesterol (LDL-C) levels between 3.3 and 4.9mmol/l and HDL-C below 1.3mmol/l, and a total cholesterol to high-density lipoprotein cholesterol (TC:HDL-C) ratio above 5. So they were typical of people in any general practitioner's list of patients with moderate hypercholesterolaemia and a low HDL-C. The aim was to bring down the LDL-C level to below 2.9mmol/l.

Some subjects were given a statin drug (lovastatin), others a placebo. The lovastatin treatment reduced LDL-C by 25 per cent, triglyceride (TG) by 15 per cent and increased HDL-C by 6 per cent. The study was stopped early because of the far greater 'event rate' (numbers of people with heart attacks and strokes) among those taking the placebo than in those on the statin. On the statin there were 40 per cent fewer fatal and non-fatal heart attacks, 32 per cent fewer serious attacks of angina, and a 33 per cent reduction in the numbers of people needing emergency coronary artery surgery.

Women, the elderly, smokers, people with high blood pressure and with diabetes all benefited from the statin, and the improvement was seen even in those with the mildest rise in blood lipid levels.

This study showed that statins will help people with relatively mild increases in cholesterol levels and with a low HDL-C – a very common pattern of hyperlipidaemia in Britain. Whether the nation could afford prescribing statins to the many millions of people in this category is arguable!

Atorvastatin Versus Revascularization Treatments (AVERT)

The Air Force study was conducted in people with relatively mild disease and no previous signs of heart disease. AVERT looked at people in the other extreme: the 341 people who entered AVERT all had known coronary artery disease with angina. They all had angiograms that showed they had narrowing of at least one coronary artery. Then they were allocated randomly to either medical treatment with the drug atorvastatin or to angioplasty (in which a balloon-tipped catheter is used to expand the narrowed coronary segment). Angioplasty is regarded as the standard treatment for coronary artery narrowing in people with angina. It is usually highly successful and has been a great addition to our ability to treat people with angina. It is routinely used during heart attacks in specialist hospitals to prevent heart muscle damage.

Of course, angioplasty does not guarantee prevention of further attacks of angina or even full heart attacks (in which an artery is completely blocked and the area of heart muscle beyond the blockage dies). Atorvastatin turned out to be more effective than angioplasty. There were 36 per cent fewer new 'cardiac' episodes (attacks of angina or heart attacks), and the time from the start of treatment to the next event was longer for those on the atorvastatin treatment than for those who had the angioplasty. TC, LDL-C and TG levels were all lower for the people on atorvastatin than for those who had the angioplasty. There were fewer serious side-effects of treatment on atorvastatin than after angioplasty.

The authors concluded that atorvastatin may help doctors to postpone or even avoid completely angioplasty procedures in some patients with mild or moderate coronary artery disease.

Cholesterol And Recurrent Events (CARE) Study

This study, like AVERT, followed people with high LDL-C levels who also had already had heart attacks. CARE's aim was to see if a statin drug (in this case pravastatin) would prevent further heart attacks. It enrolled 4,159 patients with TCs below 6.2mmol/l and LDL-Cs of 3 to 4.5mmol/l. In other words, they would have been borderline candidates for drugs if they had not had a heart attack. Half were given pravastatin and half placebo. They were followed for five years.

Pravastatin lowered the average LDL-C level by 32 per cent, maintaining it at 2.50 to 2.52 mmol/l for the whole five years. There were 24 per cent fewer heart attacks among those on pravastatin than among those on placebo. There was also a 26 per cent fall in the need for coronary artery bypass surgery, a 23 per cent reduction in angioplasty, and a 31 per cent reduction in stroke among those taking pravastatin.

Interestingly, CARE showed that women responded to pravastatin better than men, with a bigger drop in heart attacks, strokes and the need for surgery, particularly in those with higher initial LDL-C values. It also reported one odd result, that there were more cases of non-fatal breast cancer in the women receiving the pravastatin than in those on placebo. This has not been found in any other trial of pravastatin or any other statin.

Long-term Intervention with Pravastatin in Ischaemic Disease (LIPID)

This was a massive study conducted by doctors in 87 centres in Australia and New Zealand in the 1990s. More than 9,000 patients entered the full study: they received either pravastatin or placebo. They all had coronary artery disease and had been previously admitted to hospital because of a heart attack or an attack of severe angina. Their TCs on starting the trial were between 4.0 and 7.0mmol/l, and their TG less than 5.0mmol/l. Most of the patients were already taking aspirin to prevent thrombosis and a beta-blocker for their high blood pressure or abnormal heart rhythm.

LIPID had to be stopped early, after six years, because of the obvious advantage enjoyed by the statin-treated group. The patients given pravastatin showed reductions of 18 per cent in TC, 25 per cent in LDL-C and 12 per cent in TG. There was an increase of 6 per cent in HDL-C. Linked with these changes were a 24 per cent reduction in deaths due to heart events and an overall reduction in deaths from all causes of 22 per cent. People concerned with the costs of prescribing statins to so many patients must have been reassured by the news that the statin group needed 20 per cent fewer angioplasties and bypass operations. This made the overall cost of drug treatment less than the cost of patient 'rescue' with extra heart surgery.

The Scandinavian Simvastatin Survival Study (4S)

This was one of the earlier studies of the use of statins in people with hypercholesterolaemia. It is unusual in that it concentrated on patients with total cholesterol (TC) levels between 5.5 and 8.0mmol, but excluded anyone with a triglyceride (TG) above 2.4mmol/l. For five years, 4S followed 4,444 patients allocated to either the drug simvastatin or placebo. By the end of the trial there were 34 per cent fewer major heart problems among those on simvastatin than on placebo.

4S was the first trial to relate the drop in lipid levels to the fall in risk of heart attack or stroke. For each fall of 1 per cent in TC, the risk of a major cardiac event (MCE) fell by 1.9 per cent, and a 1 per cent fall in LDL-C led to a reduction of 1.7 per cent in MCEs.

West of Scotland Coronary Prevention Study (WOSCOPS)

I must admit bias towards this study, because it was conducted in my home area and I know some of the general practitioners and the men who took part in it. But it had a peculiar result. Like the 4S study, it tried to relate any fall in lipid levels to improvements in survival.

WOSCOPS followed 6,595 men who had never had a heart attack, giving them either pravastatin or placebo. Pravastatin certainly worked: there were 36 per cent fewer severe heart events among those men on it than among those on placebo. However, the fall could not be related to changes in cholesterol levels from starting levels, nor to the cholesterol levels on treatment. The authors felt that the benefits of pravastatin were not due to reduction in LDL-C alone. They did show that the men with higher-than-average triglyceride (TG) levels (more than 1.6mmol/l) benefited more from the statin than men with higher-than-average total cholesterol levels (more than 7 mmol/l), although both groups gained substantial benefit.

This conclusion, that lowering TG levels offers considerable benefits, was supported by the Stockholm Ischaemic Heart Disease Secondary Prevention Study. In its patients whose TG was lowered by more than 30 per cent, the deaths from heart disease fell by a massive 60 per cent.

This chapter could go on and on relating the different trials of drugs in hyperlipidaemia, but enough is enough. The defence of the use of lipid-lowering agents in people with hyperlipidaemias of all types rests. All the trials showed that the benefits outweigh the risk of adverse events. However, there *are* adverse effects of lipid-lowering drugs, and they will be described next, along with the details of the various drugs and drug types used to combat hyperlipidaemia.

Which Drugs for Which Patients?

Drugs that improve blood lipid levels have been a huge success. The trials listed above are only some among many that have shown that they do what they claim to – they lower cholesterol and triglyceride levels, and in doing so they prevent deaths from heart attacks and strokes in the people most vulnerable to them.

However, the best-known of these drugs are the statins, and they may not be the correct drugs for everyone with a lipid problem. Other 'lipid-lowering' types of drug are fibrates, bile-acid sequestrants and nicotinic acid. A fifth choice, oestrogens, may be used for women after the menopause with high cholesterol and LDL-C levels.

It is probably best first to explain how these different drugs work, and then to discuss which type of lipid problem each is best for.

Statins – HMG-CoA Reductase Inhibitors

The statins in current use include atorvastatin (UK brand name Lipitor), fluvastatin (Lescol), pravastatin (Lipostat) and simvastatin (Zocor). Statins hit the headlines in 2001 when cerivastatin (Lipobay) was withdrawn after reports of unacceptably high numbers of cases of muscle pains, especially when given with fibrates.

How They Work

Statins work by blocking an enzyme, HMG-CoA reductase, which is involved in the making of cholesterol in the liver. They are most effective, therefore, in reducing low-density lipoprotein cholesterol (LDL-C), but are less effective in lowering high triglyceride (TG) levels. Nevertheless they do reduce TG by between 15 and 40 per cent, depending on the dose.

By blocking the HMG-CoA reductase enzyme, statins reduce both LDL-C and VLDL, so that they reduce blood total cholesterol and TG levels, while slightly increasing HDL-C (the 'good' cholesterol). Which one your doctor chooses to use depends a lot on his or her personal experience with this class of drugs. They are probably all similar in effect and side-effects.

Dosage

Doses range up to 80mg per day for atorvastatin, fluvastatin and simvastatin, and up to 40mg per day for pravastatin.

Side-effects

Most people tolerate statins well. The main problem concerns the muscles. A few people given statins develop pains in the muscles, often in the shoulder and upper back. If this happens to you, you should stop the drug and report the effect to your doctor. The muscle problem may be made worse (even to the extent that some of the muscle tissues are destroyed, in a process called *rhabdomyolysis*) if the drug is given with fibrates, which are mainly used to lower TG levels. The problem may also be made worse if you are taking drugs for other illnesses, such as cyclosporin (to prevent transplant rejection), the antibiotic erythromycin, and the antifungal ketoconazole.

Other less often reported side-effects include headache, abdominal pain, flatulence, diarrhoea, nausea and vomiting. There have been very rare reports of rashes and allergic reactions to statins. Statins combine well with bile-acid sequestrants, but must be used with great care with fibrates or nicotinic acid.

You will not be prescribed statins if you have liver disease or are a heavy drinker, as they can be toxic (poisonous) to a liver that is showing chronic disease, such as active hepatitis or alcoholic degeneration. Your doctor will take blood for liver function tests before you start on a statin, and repeat the tests every six months.

Fibrates

Fibrates include bezafibrate (Bezalip), ciprofibrate (Modalim), fenofibrate (Lipantil) and gemfibrozil (Lopid).

How They Work
Fibrates lower VLDL by blocking its synthesis in the liver, so they are useful in treating combined hypercholesterolaemia and hypertriglyceridaemia. They may also stimulate the clearance of excess LDL-C from the plasma. Gemfibrozil is thought to be the most effective in treating the Fredrickson type 5 form of high VLDL dyslipidaemia, and the others have a reputation for being better than gemfibrozil at lowering LDL-C levels. All fibrates tend to raise HDL-C, but only by a small amount.

Dosage
Bezafibrate is given as 200mg three times daily, or as a slow-release preparation of 400mg once daily. Ciprofibrate is given as a single daily 100-mg dose. Fenofibrate is given either as 100mg three times daily or a 200-mg slow-release tablet once daily. Gemfibrozil has a dose of 600mg twice daily.

Side-effects

Like the statins, most people have no trouble taking the fibrates. However, there are some reports of nausea, diarrhoea, gallstones, alopecia and muscle weakness with fibrates, and your doctor will wish to monitor your liver regularly. There are rare cases of liver upsets on fibrates.

Very great care must be taken if you are considering taking a fibrate with a statin, as the combination can lead to muscle problems. However, there are few problems in prescribing fibrates along with nicotinic acid or bile acid sequestrants.

Bile-acid Sequestrants

There are two current bile-acid sequestrants: cholestyramine (Questran) and colestipol (Colestid).

How They Work

Bile-acid sequestrants work by 'binding' to the bile acids in the gut, so that they can no longer deliver fats to the liver for processing into new cholesterol and triglyceride. The liver therefore needs to 'suck' cholesterol back into it from the circulation. This sets up a flow of fats from their deposits in the endothelium through the circulation into the liver. Plasma cholesterol levels therefore fall. However, there may be a downside – VLDL-C and TG levels may rise.

Cholestyramine and colestipol are used in people with raised LDL-C, but not raised TG levels – the Fredrickson type 2a hyperlipidaemia. They are not used in hypertriglyceridaemia, where there is a problem with beta-lipoprotein, or in people with constipation.

Side-effects

In fact, constipation is the main side-effect of bile-acid sequestrants, and may be too inconvenient for people to continue with them, although it is usually relieved by taking 'bulking' laxatives such as Fybogel.

Bile-acid sequestrants may reduce the absorption of other important drugs, making them less effective. They are therefore not usually given within three hours of taking doses of warfarin (to stop blood-clotting), thyroxine (thyroid hormone), diuretics, and beta-blockers (usually given for high blood pressure, but sometimes for an abnormal heart rhythm). They may also affect the uptake from the gut of folic acid (given before and during pregnancy, mainly to prevent spina bifida and other spine and brain abnormalities in the developing foetus) and vitamins A and D.

People taking bile-acid sequestrants should have their blood monitored for possible malabsorption problems (such as anaemia) each year. They can be given with each of the other lipid-lowering drug types.

Nicotinic Acid

Nicotinic acid is a vitamin, but the dose used to lower blood lipid levels is much higher than the usual daily requirement for this nutrient.

How It Works

Nicotinic acid reduces the formation of VLDL in the liver, at the same time reducing the level of free fatty acids (the 'building blocks' of cholesterol) in the circulation. It also blocks the production of apolipoprotein B, thereby lowering its level in the blood.

Nicotinic acid is used for all the Fredrickson hyperlipidaemia types except type 1. It decreases VLDL-C and LDL-C, while increasing HDL-C by a very substantial 15 to 25 per cent. It is the only lipid-lowering drug to substantially decrease blood lipoprotein(a) levels.

Dosage

It is given either three times daily, starting with doses of around 100 to 250mg, then rising gradually to as much as 4.5 to 6 grams daily. There are sustained-release preparations to provide up to 2 grams daily, but higher doses than that may cause liver problems.

Side-effects

The main problem with nicotinic acid is flushing, which can be reduced by taking an aspirin about 15 to 30 minutes beforehand. Nicotinic acid can add to the effect of blood pressure-lowering drugs, so you should be warned about that. It can cause gout, a skin condition called *acanthosis nigricans* and swelling of the retina in the back of the eye, but happily all these disappear when the drug is stopped.

People with active liver disease, diabetes (nicotinic acid can raise blood glucose levels) and gout should probably not take nicotinic acid. If you are taking it, you should have a blood test to check your liver and blood glucose every six months or so.

It can be given safely with fibrates and bile-acid sequestrants, but not with statins, as it may increase the risk of severe muscle reactions. High doses may cause a form of hepatitis that can be severe (with tenderness in the upper right abdomen, nausea, weakness and jaundice), but this reverses when the drug is stopped.

Oestrogens

Oestrogens given in the usual dose for hormone replacement therapy (HRT) decrease LDL-C by 10 to 15 per cent and increase HDL-C by 15 to 25 per cent in older women with the Fredrickson type 2a form of hypercholesterolaemia. Patients should follow the rule (to protect the womb from cancer) of having a combined oestrogen/progestogen pill if they have not had a hysterectomy. However, this causes the plasma TG to rise by between 5 and 10 per cent, so there is a mixed response to the drug.

The problem with this strategy is that there has been no published evidence that giving HRT to postmenopausal women with hyperlipidaemia actually protects them against heart attacks or strokes. Women who already have hypertriglyceridaemia should not take oestrogens, as they cause the TG to rise even further, in theory raising their risks of heart disease.

So HRT should be considered as a choice for older women with hypercholesterolaemia with no contraindications to oestrogens and who accept the principle of HRT. Women taking HRT should have their blood lipid profile performed every six months, and should have their breasts examined at the same time. Some experts recommend an annual mammogram for these women: this seems to me to be a little extreme. Oestrogens can be safely used along with the other lipid-lowering drugs.

Selecting the Right Drug for the Patient and Type of Lipid Problem

Reading through the actions and drawbacks of the various drugs for lowering cholesterol and triglyceride levels, it would be surprising if you were not a little confused about who should be given what. Here I am indebted to a summary written by Drs L A Carlson, A M Gotto and D R Illingworth, in a *Science Press Review of Current Hyperlipidaemia* in 2000. These experts write the following:

For primary prevention of heart disease
(in people with hyperlipidaemia but no heart or other disease of the circulation to date)

- *Bile-acid sequestrants are preferred if the patient is younger and at low risk.*
- *Statins are preferred for high risk patients or those with severe hypercholesterolaemia who need their LDL-C lowered substantially.*
- *Nicotinic acid is beneficial for such patients, though they often find they cannot tolerate its side-effects.*
- *Fibrates have the disadvantage in this group of people of possibly actually raising LDL-C in a small proportion of them.*

In combined hyperlipidaemia, in which both TG and LDL-C are raised

- *Nicotinic acid and fibrates are the first choice, because of their dual action on both types of lipid.*
- *The statins are alternatives to nicotinic acid when patients cannot tolerate it, as they do have some effect on triglycerides.*

For hypertriglyceridaemia

- *Fibrates and nicotinic acid are the choice for hypertriglyceridaemia. However, if the patient also has diabetes (a high TG is common in diabetes), nicotinic acid should not be given as it can disturb the glucose control. In Fredrickson type 5 hyperlipidaemia, in which there can be repeated attacks of pancreatitis, then nicotinic acid is the choice.*

For people with low HDL-C and no other lipid problem

● *Nicotinic acid or fibrate treatment might be considered to raise it.*

Chapter Eight

Other Treatments and Controversies

Antioxidants

Studies suggesting that the oxidisation (a process where exposure to oxygen causes damage, as when metal rusts or a chopped apple left out in the open goes brown) of low-density lipoprotein (LDL) particles inside the plaques of atheroma in the artery walls is the underlying cause of heart attacks and strokes have led to many studies of the use of antioxidants such as vitamin E in people with hyperlipidaemias. These studies have been backed up by the Nurses Health Study and the Health Professionals Follow-Up Study, in both of which the people with the highest levels of vitamin E in their blood had the lowest rates of coronary disease. Their blood vitamin E levels were in fact so high that they must have been taking it as a vitamin supplement, and not just from the food they were eating.

The same studies showed that two other popular antioxidants, vitamin C and beta-carotene, had no effect on coronary disease in non-smokers. In fact, beta-carotene may even do harm. In two studies (the Coronary Angioplasty and Rotablator Atherectomy Trial, or CARAT; and the Alpha-Tocopherol/Beta-carotene Trial, or ATBC), beta-carotene was linked to an increase in heart deaths.

So there is no reason to try to improve your chances of avoiding a heart attack or stroke by taking either beta-carotene or vitamin C, but there may be some value in taking vitamin E. The trials to prove or disprove this are still going on. Until they are finished there is probably no good reason to take any antioxidant as a treatment for hyperlipidaemia.

Omega-3 Fatty Acids

Omega-3 fatty acids, made from fish oils, have been shown to reduce TG levels. They may be used if other treatments are not successful. However, it is too soon to know how safe they are over many years.

They may cause bleeding, so should not be used along with anticoagulants or by people with bleeding problems. And one strange fact stressed by Drs Carlson, Gotto and Illingworth is that some fish-oil capsules actually contain cholesterol, which tends to negate their beneficial effects!

Other Nutrients

For completeness, I must mention here the vitamins folic acid, B6 (pyridoxine) and B12 (cyanocobalamin), and their effect on the substance homocysteine.

We may hear a lot more about homocysteine in the next few years. Homocysteine is an 'amino-acid', one of the 'building blocks' of proteins fundamental to the chemistry of all the cells of our bodies. Every cell nucleus (the powerhouse of every living cell) is made up of specialised proteins, which also form the structure of muscles. Homocysteine is just one of many amino-acids used to make them.

Until recently, homocysteine was looked upon as just another amino-acid that we get from food and that we need, just like all the others, for healthy organs and tissues. Now there is concern about it. High levels of homocysteine in the blood have been linked, just as clearly as high levels of lipids, to rapidly advancing atheroma and early deaths due to heart disease and strokes. It is suggested that too high a level of homocysteine in the blood damages the endothelium, so that it cannot produce the muscle-relaxing series of chemicals that open up the arteries. The result is not only narrowed arteries, but a damaged endothelium and advanced atheroma. So the combination of a high cholesterol and a high homocysteine level may be lethal.

This idea has been supported by a study of 587 people with known coronary artery disease whose blood homocysteine levels were measured. They were divided up into three groups: those with levels under 15mmol/l, those with levels between 15 and 19mmol/l, and those with levels of 20mmol/l or more. Over the next four years there were nearly three times the deaths in the second group, and four and a half times the deaths in the third group, than in the first.

It is one thing to say that the higher your homocysteine level, the higher the risk that you will die early from a heart attack, but another to say that lowering your homocysteine will reduce that risk. However, it does seem reasonable to suggest that if your homocysteine level is higher than normal (say over 16mmol/l), it may help if you try to reduce it.

Happily, this can be achieved fairly easily and safely by taking just a small amount of the vitamin folic acid in a dose of 1 or 2mg per day. If that does not lower your homocysteine level, you can try taking pyridoxine (vitamin B6) 25mg per day. There is no need to take a higher dose.

A Word of Warning

If you are about to take either folic acid or pyridoxine, you should have your blood levels of vitamin B12 measured first. This is because a very small number of people may have early pernicious anaemia, a condition in which the stomach is unable to digest vitamin B12, so that there is a B12 deficiency in the blood. This leads to a particular form of anaemia, because the bone marrow needs B12 to form red blood cells correctly. In such people, taking folic acid can worsen the condition, and particularly the nerve symptoms that appear along with the anaemia.

Chapter Nine

Some Familiar Stories

Until now, most of the book has dealt with the science of cholesterol, how when it is too high it harms our blood vessels, and how it can be treated. It has not brought you personally into the picture, so it may be difficult to relate your own story to what you have read up to this point. So this chapter is a series of descriptions of patients I have met over the years who have needed treatment to bring down their raised cholesterol levels. You may well recognise yourself in one of these stories.

The Wilson Family

In the 1960s, when I was starting out in my medical career, doctors like myself knew very little about the hyperlipidaemias, and even less about how to treat them. I got my training in them early, however, as I had a family in my practice who knew only too well how lethal they could be.

My first meeting with a member of this family was to attend a 34-year-old man with chest pains. He was obviously having a severe heart attack, and despite all our efforts he died that night, only a few hours after his admission to hospital. The family were as philosophical as they could be under the tragic circumstances. They had seen all too many of their fathers, uncles, brothers and cousins die in exactly the same way before they reached 40.

I was astonished at this, and informed our local heart specialist about the family. He was glad to investigate, and found huge levels of total cholesterol and triglycerides in virtually every family member. They were not obese, they worked very hard – most of the men were fishermen, probably the hardest physical job of all – and they did not smoke. Nor did they have high blood pressure. They had true primary hyperlipidaemia, and this was enough to cause their early deaths. Even the women in the family were affected, although they had their heart attacks, on average, around 10 years later than their menfolk.

In the late 1960s and early 1970s all we could do to help them was to put them on a strict very low-fat diet. We later got wiser and added in fish oils. Funnily enough, fishermen rarely eat fish. They were often knee-deep in the very food that could have prolonged their lives – herring – but they preferred bacon and eggs. Changing how they ate did help a little, but it was only after we were able to prescribe lipid-lowering drugs that we really made a difference to the family. Now all of them, even the teenagers, are on a combination of a statin and a fibrate, and their lipid levels are near normal. For the first time the men are living into their 70s, and they (and their doctors) are very grateful.

That family was difficult to diagnose, because their high blood cholesterol levels did not produce any outward signs: they had no fatty lumps in their skin, they did not look yellow, they did not have 'senile arcs' around their irises. But their artery walls were full of fat, and their coronaries were the worst affected of all.

Their pattern of illness is relatively rare, and the numbers of early deaths were very high, but it is a lesson for others with an incidental finding, say at an insurance medical, of a high cholesterol. If this describes you, then look back to your family history. Did your father, or uncles, grandfathers, or even women relatives die early from heart disease? If they did, that is a powerful reason for taking extra care of your own cholesterol levels. You are lucky enough to live in an age when, with modern management, you can add 30 or more active and healthy years to your lifespan.

Most people with a high cholesterol level, however, don't have such a daunting family history of early death. The typical case is a relatively young man (less often a woman) who is found to have abnormally high blood lipid levels at a routine medical. It may be at a 'well man' clinic, which most men in their 40s are asked to attend by their family doctors, at least in Britain. Most people attending such clinics are, by definition (because they are picked out from their doctors' lists as not having been seen for some time) well. So they tend not to have any symptoms, or if they have had them, they have not considered them serious enough to see their doctor about.

Take Bill, for example. He is a 47-year old salesman, too busy to have health check-ups, who only attended when persuaded to do so by his wife, who was tired of explaining to their doctor why he hadn't kept the last two well-man clinic appointments. Bill wasn't surprised to find that he had a high cholesterol (TC was 8.2mmol/l). He ate a lot 'on the hoof' at fast food restaurants and in hotels, and loved his chips. And he was two stones overweight.

The lack of surprise went with lack of concern, too. He felt well, and he didn't see how he could alter his lifestyle at the moment. He was at a crucial point in his career, and any change might rock the boat, just when he was in line for an area manager's job. So he didn't return for the follow-up visit, when he was to see the practice dietician and get more lifestyle advice. Despite three more letters, he couldn't find the time to attend the surgery.

Four months later, Bill suffered his first bout of chest pain. He had had a particularly heavy lunch – in fact to celebrate that manager's job at last. While tucking into the sweet course, this dull ache appeared just to the left of the centre of his chest. It spread to his back, and up into the left side of his jaw. He had to stop eating, and sat back in his chair, panic rising as the pain intensified.

He was very lucky in two ways that day. He was with Sue, his wife, who was a nurse and recognised the signs. And Sue knew that the best immediate treatment was a whole adult-strength aspirin (a 300-milligram dose). She also knew that she had to get him as fast as possible to the local hospital, which was only five minutes away. So without fuss she drove him there, where he was given an intravenous clot-busting drug (thrombokinase) and admitted to the heart unit. (For more about aspirin, see Chapter Fourteen.)

The fast treatment ensured that Bill's impending 'heart attack' was arrested before it damaged his heart muscle irrevocably. An electrocardiogram (ECG) showed that he had severe angina (pain in the chest due to lack of oxygen supply to the heart muscle) but not a full 'infarction' (loss of heart muscle due to complete blockage of the blood flow in the coronary arteries.)

Bill's pain came as a shock to him. It has to be said here that most people, when they first get a pain like this while eating, put it down to 'indigestion' and take an antacid for a while. That can be a big mistake, because every minute matters if you are to prevent permanent damage to your heart. Luckily Bill did not make that mistake.

Nor did he continue to make his other mistake – of ignoring the high cholesterol. From that time on, Bill has been sticking to a much healthier lifestyle, taking a statin and a daily low-dose aspirin (75mg), and is delegating a lot of his work to his assistants. Sue is delighted, and looks upon that first episode of angina as a life-saver. He has lost weight, and is feeling much fitter than he was.

Bill had a coronary angiogram (an X-ray which shows the coronary arteries in outline) in that first admission to hospital. He was told that it showed he had atheroma, with narrowing in all three coronary arteries, and that he might need bypass or angioplasty surgery in the future. However, he has done so well in the year that has passed, with no more angina episodes, that a repeat angiogram has shown less coronary narrowing. In fact, the circulation to his heart muscle is improving thanks to his new lifestyle and drugs. He now has the same attitude to the health of his heart as to his work, and he won't backslide. He probably will never need cardiac surgery.

Arthur

Arthur wasn't as lucky as Bill. At 56, he had never been ill. A city taxi driver working odd hours – one week night shift, another week on afternoons and evenings – he never had time to visit his doctor, and hadn't attended any of the invitations to attend for a well-man examination. So when he had his heart attack, while he was driving, he had no one with him to slip him an aspirin. A colleague saw him stopped by the side of the road, saw how unwell he looked, and took him straight to the local Accident and Emergency Department.

There the doctors gave Arthur an aspirin and an injection of the clot-busting drug thrombokinase, and arranged for an emergency coronary angiogram. It showed severe atheroma, with narrowing of all three coronary arteries, and because the ECG showed his heart was seriously short of oxygen, he had an emergency triple bypass operation.

From then on, Arthur did remarkably well. He recovered quickly from the operation, his chest pain disappeared and his ECG improved. The bypasses had worked well. But his doctors stressed to him that his life had to change. He had a total cholesterol of more than 9mmol/l.

Because his heart muscle showed some residual damage, he was put on aspirin and warfarin to prevent further clots (see Chapter Ten), and introduced to the hospital dietician for advice on how to eat more healthily. He was counselled, too, on his job. After a heart attack there is a higher than normal risk of having a second one. Even though Arthur was taking all the precautions he could to prevent a further attack, his doctors suggested that he stop driving for a living. Luckily his taxi firm needed a man in the office to organise calls – and Arthur was the natural choice. His employers were asked, too, to give him a regular timetable, without shift changes. It is very difficult to eat wisely when your working hours are erratic and vary from week to week. Arthur didn't much like the change, but he put up with it, and a year later he is fit and well. Three evenings a week he takes his grandsons to a sports centre, where they swim and he 'works out' with exercises devised specially for him by the physiotherapists from the hospital heart department.

Michael

I'm not sure whether there really is such a thing as 'an addictive personality', defined as a person who has inherited a tendency to become addicted to whatever is the trendy drug or habit of the day. The psychiatrists argue a lot about whether addiction is inborn or is due to circumstances in early life. Whichever the cause (and I might admit to there being a bit of both in most addicts), Michael was certainly an addict.

He was addicted to drink, to the extent that he drank between four and eight strong ales (those 'Special Brews' that contain more than 10 per cent alcohol) a day, and he was addicted to tobacco, in that he admitted to smoking around 30 cigarettes a day. I suspect his real cigarette load was closer to 60.

At 45 he had made his money in business deals abroad, and had retired. I suspect here, too, that he had been forced to retire, with a 'golden handshake', largely because of his drinking. Trouble with the law (drink driving) and with Jean, his wife (his inability to remain sober, and his impotence) led him to seek advice.

He got it in no uncertain terms. He was shown the results of his liver tests, and warned that he faced liver failure within a year or two unless he stopped all alcohol. But the surprise for us was that he also had a very high total cholesterol level, of around 9mmol/l, and a triglyceride of 3mmol/l. We were surprised because people who drink a lot often have relatively low blood lipid levels.

Give Michael his due, he took our advice. He did stop drinking and even his smoking, and he changed his lifestyle. He got his appetite back, and started eating more healthily, and for a while everything looked good. However, his total cholesterol level climbed even higher, to over 10mmol/l. He was started on a statin drug, which rapidly lowered it again, though not without a period of muscle pain that nearly led to him stopping the drug.

Now Michael is on the wagon permanently, as far as we can see. He is taking his statin every day, his liver function tests are much better, and he is far healthier. However, there has been one semi-drawback to bringing him back to sobriety and health. He has become a lay preacher and a public campaigner against strong drink and cigarettes. He has become so addicted to these causes that Jean has left home. She says she preferred her drunken old husband to this intolerant new one. We can't win them all.

Jenny

Jenny would be the first to admit she is overweight. At 38 she has been overweight since she was in her teens. Not that it bothers her too much. She is a cheerful, bubbly woman who brightens everyone up in her work caring for adults with learning difficulties. And she is happily married to her equally pleasant husband. They do have one sadness, however. They have never been able to have children. Her periods were always erratic, and she was finally given the diagnosis of polycystic ovarian syndrome (PCOS) two years ago, when she eventually asked for help in conceiving.

Sadly she had left it too late. In polycystic ovarian syndrome there are several obstacles to conception, the main one being the inability of the ovaries to 'drop' an egg once a month into her womb. She was already into an early menopause by the time she had sought help.

However, that consultation with her doctor about her infertility produced other test results that needed serious discussion. It turned out that she had high blood pressure, a high fasting blood glucose level, a high insulin level, and very high cholesterol (12mmol/l). This combination of obesity (she was apple-shaped, with a lot of extra weight around her waist), high blood pressure, a tendency to diabetes (high glucose) with 'insulin resistance' (the high insulin), and high blood lipids has been given the title of 'syndrome X'.

This is not the place to go into syndrome X in detail. If you have it, you might like to read about it in How to Cope Successfully with Diabetes, another book in the Wellhouse series. It is enough to state here that people with syndrome X are at much higher risk of early heart attacks and strokes than are the rest of the population. They must attend to all the aspects of their condition, to make sure that their blood pressure and blood glucose levels are brought down into the normal range. They can do that by losing their excess weight, by healthier eating and more exercise. That should also lower their high cholesterol levels, which should be checked at least every six months. If it doesn't, they should also take a statin or fibrate drug, depending on the pattern of the blood lipid levels.

This was put to Jenny, in a straightforward, and hopefully not frightening way. She remembered a maiden aunt who had been obese, had developed diabetes in her 40s, and had a heart attack at 50, and did not want to follow in her footsteps. So she took the advice very seriously. She joined a weight-loss programme and bought a dog to walk every evening, so that she would be forced to exercise more. She was put on an 'ACE inhibitor' drug to lower her blood pressure and to help her kidneys, which were 'leaking' a tiny amount of protein. This is a sign that they are in early trouble from the effects of high blood pressure. Jenny also arranged for a monthly appointment to monitor her blood pressure and a three-monthly appointment to test her blood lipids.

Six months later, her doctor could hardly recognise her. Three stones lighter, Jenny's blood pressure and blood glucose levels were normal, and her total cholesterol was 6mmol/l. If she remains this well, she will probably not develop the diabetes that had been predicted for her. She had even had three normal periods, so that the early menopause diagnosis may have been wrong. She is even thinking again of perhaps a last try at motherhood. She has not yet been started on a lipid-lowering drug, but she will be watched through the next few years to make sure that the cholesterol levels don't start to rise again. If they do, she will be started on a statin without hesitation.

Anne

Anne was 24 when she had her first warning sign that she might be prone to diabetes. A routine urine test during her first pregnancy tested positive for glucose. She was asked to give blood the next morning before she had breakfast, so that there was a gap of 12 hours between her last meal and the sample. It showed a higher than normal amount of glucose (around 6mmol/l). She was sent to a team specialising in 'gestational diabetes' (diabetes that starts during pregnancy), who gave her advice on how to eat more healthily and to exercise (she was two stones overweight).

She obeyed the rules, lost her excess weight, and eventually had a healthy daughter weighing over 8 pounds at birth. Six weeks later at her post-natal visit, Anne had a normal blood glucose level of 4mmol/l, and was told that the threat of diabetes had passed. She carried on with her life as usual, and forgot about her brush with her high blood glucose.

However, she also forgot about the healthy diet and the exercise. Ten years later she was back to being nearly three stones overweight. She began to feel sleepier than normal during the day, she became thirsty, and she was tired all the time. Her husband persuaded her to see her doctor, who quickly found that her diabetes had come back. This time it was a permanent change. Despite her reverting back to her healthier lifestyle, and losing the extra weight, Anne's blood glucose levels remained too high for comfort, and her doctor started her on glucose-lowering medicines.

Diabetes does not often arrive on its own in women. It comes with complications, one of which is often a high triglyceride (TG) level. This was the case with Anne. Blood lipid profiles are always performed in every newly diagnosed case of diabetes, and Anne's were abnormal enough to talk seriously with her about her eating habits and lifestyle. She had a total cholesterol of 9mmol/l, and a TG level of 3.5mmol/l, which together presented a serious risk of heart attack or stroke.

So she had to cope with two new diagnoses – her diabetes and her high cholesterol. She did well initially, losing weight and getting fitter with a combination of better eating and more exercise. Her daughter, now 10 years old, had found an aptitude for ice-skating, and Anne took great delight in joining her at the local rink as often as they could. She started feeling much better, but her TG remained obstinately high, at over 3.5mmol/l. Her doctor started her on a fibrate and her TG fell to below 1.5mmol/l. This was considered satisfactory, and she has remained on it ever since, although she admits to failing to notice any difference in well-being after the drop.

This is one of the problems in having to take drugs to lower cholesterol or triglyceride levels: people don't feel any immediate or even long-term advantage in taking them. The advantages are only really seen in the statistics, which show that taking them reduces risks of heart attacks and strokes in years to come. It is sometimes difficult to persuade people that the nuisance of taking a drug every day is worth the reduction of a risk of something which might not happen anyway.

Christine

Christine didn't like the idea of the menopause, but at 50 she was staring hers in the face. So she opted for hormone replacement therapy (HRT), which suited her beautifully. The combination of the two hormones, oestrogen and progestogen, kept her hot flushes at bay, helped her to feel good, and improved her sex life. So she wanted to keep on taking it for as long as possible. Her doctor, however, was aware that HRT sometimes raises TG levels, so she monitored them over the first two to three years. Sure enough, Christine's TG level slowly climbed from her original figure of 1.5mmol/l to 3mmol/l, a level at which her doctor became concerned. On the positive side, her total cholesterol had dropped from 6.8mmol/l to 6.2mmol/l, with most of the drop being due to a fall in LDL-C. This good result still left her with a high TC and TG.

It left her doctor in a quandary. The big rise in TG was an unwanted change, the bad effects of which might outweigh the relatively small fall in TC. Was the HRT putting Christine at a higher risk of a heart attack? If so, should it be stopped, or should she be given a lipid-lowering drug on top of her HRT? It is not normally good medical practice to add a second drug to counteract the bad effects of a first one, but Christine was given the option by her doctor, and decided to choose the HRT/lipid-lowering combination.

It worked for her. Her TC and TG both dropped further, to 4.7mmol/l and 0.9mmol/l respectively. These were considered excellent results and a huge reduction in heart risk, and she is continuing to take both HRT and a fibrate. She is very happy with her life.

Peter

Peter, at 58, a secondary schoolteacher, was pushed into having a medical by his wife. He didn't think it was at all necessary to see his doctor, as he had not had a day off work for 20 years and 'didn't feel any different from when he was in his thirties'. So he went only to please her, and expected to sail through the medical.

He didn't sail through it. His total cholesterol (TC) was 8.2mmol/l. Everything else was normal – his blood pressure, his fasting blood glucose, his ECG, and even his exercise ECG (he was put on a treadmill and asked to walk at increasing speeds, up increasing slopes, while connected to the ECG machine) were all normal. Asked about his eating habits, he admitted to a liking for the occasional 'fry-up', but on the whole he ate healthily, with plenty of fruit and vegetables, and took plenty of exercise. He wasn't overweight.

These results left his doctors in a quandary. Should they try to lower his cholesterol level even though it had not yet done any obvious harm? Or should they just forget about it, and let him carry on as he was? They looked in more detail at his lipid levels. Within the TC figure of 8.2mmol/l, his LDL-C level was 6.8mmol/l. This left only 1.4mmol/l for HDL-C. To complicate things further, his TG (triglyceride) level was 4.5mmol/l.

With this pattern of a high LDL-C and TG and a relatively low HDL-C, Peter's doctors calculated that he was at too high a risk of a sudden heart attack to ignore. They assumed (because of his satisfactory lifestyle) that he had a 'primary' hyperlipidaemia (in that he had inherited his abnormal lipid profile), so they started him on a statin drug to take once a day. Peter wasn't so sure about taking it, because he felt so well. His doctors decided to let him weigh up the evidence for lowering his blood lipids for himself, and showed him the results of the WOSCOPS study, along with the others mentioned in Chapter Seven. When his wife reminded him of his father's death at 60 from an unexpected heart attack, Peter accepted the evidence and started on the statin drug.

Now, two years later, Peter has a TC of 4.8mmol/l, an LDL-C of 3.0 and an HDL-C of 1.8. His TG level has also fallen, to 1.8mmol/l. His doctors and, more importantly, his wife, are satisfied with these figures. He doesn't feel any better than he did before he started on his treatment, but that is not surprising because he felt perfectly well then. But he is now older than his father was when he died, and he looks on that as a milestone. His mother is still alive at 84: he is aiming to follow in her footsteps.

Moira

Moira, at 45, has had high blood pressure since her first pregnancy at the age of 24. It was discovered when she went for her first ante-natal check. So for 21 years she has had to have regular blood-pressure checks. Her drugs have always kept her blood pressure under reasonably good control, but she has had to change them over the years.

Doctors have a host of blood pressure-lowering drugs from which to choose. They act in different ways, and what suits some people may not suit others. This turned out to be the case for Moira. Most people who have been newly found to have high blood pressure are given a standard mixture of two types of drug – a 'diuretic' and a 'beta-blocker'. The diuretic acts on the kidneys, so that they become more active in removing salt and water from the body. This lowers blood pressure by reducing the volume of fluid that the heart has to pump round the body. Beta-blockers work by slowing the rate at which the heart beats and reducing the force with which it beats. The two types of drug are complementary, and are usually very effective.

They certainly kept Moira's blood pressure under control, but they had a side-effect of which she was completely unaware. They tended to raise her total cholesterol (mainly the LDL-C) and her TG level. Her doctors decided to change her prescription, so that she would now have a drug that would at least not worsen her lipid profile and might even lower the TC and TG levels. So they switched her to an 'ACE inhibitor', a drug that interferes with the chemical 'message' (called the renin-angiotensin system) which the kidney sends to the heart to make it beat more strongly and faster.

The switch worked. Moira's blood pressure was kept under good control, and her lipid profile returned to less risky levels. Her LDL-C and TG fell, and her HDL-C rose slightly. Bringing down her blood pressure and her LDL-C and TG levels together steeply improved her chances of avoiding a heart attack and stroke, but her doctors felt that they could do more. The TG remained higher, proportionately, than her LDL-C, so they decided to offer her long-term treatment with a fibrate, on top of her ACE-inhibitor.

Moira now has TC, LDL-C and TG levels all within the normal range, and so far she has had no serious side-effects from her blood pressure-lowering or her lipid-lowering drugs. She understands that she will have to have her pressure checked every month, and her lipids checked at least every year, for the rest of her life. Hopefully that will be a much longer time than she could have expected without them.

James Fixx

All the case histories in this chapter so far are success stories. That is deliberate, because I want the book to be optimistic. If you identify with one of them, you can use it as an example to follow. However, there isn't always such a happy ending.

The American James Fixx wrote his book *The Complete Book of Running* in 1977. He was probably the person most responsible for popularising running, or jogging, as a sport for everyone. When he was in his thirties, he lived the life of a couch potato. He weighed 100kg (around 16 stones) and was breathless when he tried to run only 50 metres.

He took up running, and in 10 years he lost 25kg (around 4 stones), had run the equivalent of once around the Equator, had completed many marathons, and was running 16 kilometres (10 miles) every day. By 1984, doctors all over the world were recommending his book to everyone who needed to become fit, and to help their hearts. Runners looked on Mr Fixx's book as the bible of good health.

Then he died, of a heart attack, while running. By this time he was in his late fifties. What Mr Fixx had not understood was that exercise might be a good thing, but it was certainly not everything. He did not know that there are times when you need help other than exercise.

At the post-mortem it was found that he had severe atheroma, affecting all his coronary arteries. Much of the fat in his arteries was probably laid down during his obese, under-exercised period. It may also have been inherited, as he had written that his father had died in his 30s from coronary artery disease. We don't know for sure, however, because nowhere in his book on running does he mention having had any blood tests for cholesterol or other fats.

It is clear, with hindsight, that Fixx thought he could 'run through' his coronary pain, and that he felt he could keep his heart going by exercising more, rather than less. In fact, running for him was an obsession. Perhaps if he had asked for medical advice he would have lived a lot longer. Informed about his high risk from atheroma, he could have used all the methods described in this book to keep his blood lipids in the right range, including drugs to lower them, and two days of rest a week from his punishing training schedule.

Of course, the James Fixx story could still be looked upon as a success. He did enjoy 20 years of life after starting on his running career, and the chances are that he would have died much earlier if he had remained an overweight couch potato. But the suspicion remains that if he had looked at his health problems from a 'total risk-management' point of view, he may well have lived longer still. The next chapter describes this total risk-management regimen, and how anyone can follow it. It puts cholesterol and the other lipids in their place in relationship to other aspects of healthy living and protecting your heart and brain.

Chapter Ten

Lowering the Risks – Your Total Risk Management Programme

Maybe the title of this book is a little misleading. After all, its prime aim is not to help you lower your cholesterol levels. It is to help you avoid premature death and disability from a heart attack or stroke. Coping with cholesterol is only part of what you need to do to reduce your risk of one of these two very common catastrophes, which kill more than half of the populations of developed countries today.

Having read this far, you will already know that besides a high cholesterol, the other main risks to your heart and brain are smoking, high blood pressure, diabetes, lack of exercise and obesity. Other things that put you at risk of a heart attack or stroke are being male and being old, but you can do nothing about either of them.

Calculating Your Risk

In the 1990s, the data from the Framingham studies mentioned in Chapter Three were brought together to form a series of 'tables of coronary risk'. That is, charts from which you can calculate your risk of having a coronary thrombosis (a fatal or disabling heart attack) within the next 10 years. All you need to know to work out your own risk is your gender, age, blood pressure (the 'systolic', or higher, reading), total cholesterol level, whether or not you smoke, and whether or not you have diabetes.

There are eight charts in all, four for men and four for women. The four charts for each sex comprise separate ones for smokers and non-smokers, and for people with diabetes who smoke or don't smoke. They are also divided by age, from 30, in 10-year spans up to 70, so that within each of the four groups of charts, there are five sub-charts. On the upright axis are rising blood pressure levels, and on the horizontal axis are the cholesterol levels. All these help you to identify your own place on the chart.

The tables reproduced here are adapted from the Framingham data, and versions of them are used by every general practitioner.

MEN
Risk of coronary heart disease

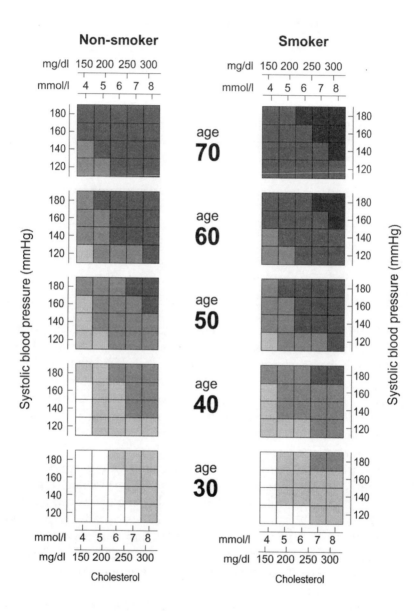

MEN WITH DIABETES
Risk of coronary heart disease

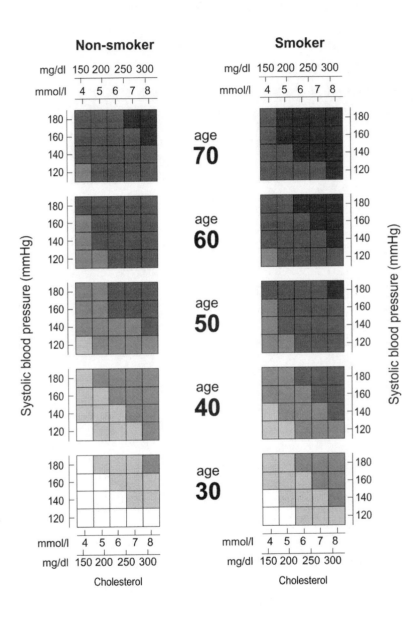

WOMEN
Risk of coronary heart disease

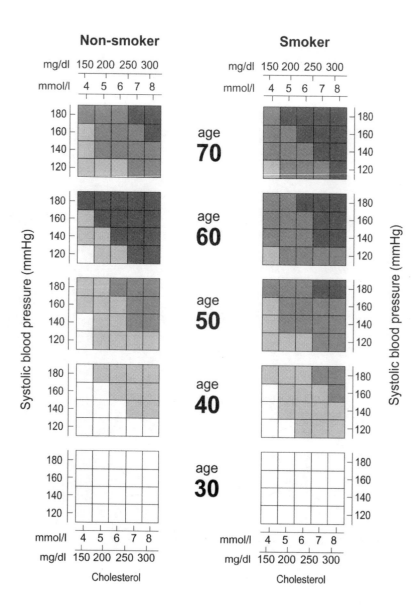

Non-smoker

Smoker

Systolic blood pressure (mmHg)

Cholesterol

WOMEN WITH DIABETES
Risk of coronary heart disease

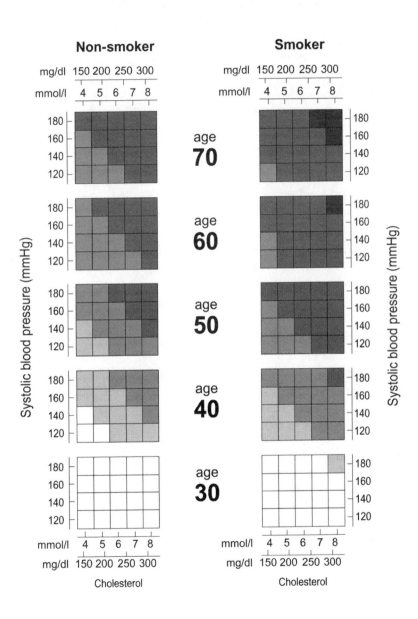

If you know your total cholesterol and blood pressure levels (presumably you know your age, sex and whether or not you have diabetes!), you can work out how high your risk is. You will fit into one of these boxes: find the box, and read off your risk. It will range from under 5 per cent to over 40 per cent in the next five years.

Once you have done this, you can see how you can lower the risk. By stopping smoking, you move from one more dangerous chart to another less dangerous one. By reducing your blood pressure or total cholesterol, you move from nearer the top right corner towards the bottom left, reducing your risk accordingly.

These charts were compiled from American data, so they may not be absolutely accurate as a guide to the chance of a heart attack in the populations of Britain and other European countries. However, they will not be far out. They are certainly close enough to show that if you can move from a box that is more to the right and the top of the chart into a box that is more to the left and the bottom, you will improve your chances of keeping healthier longer. You can even calculate by how much you are reducing your heart attack risk – and that can be a big incentive to continuing with your new lifestyle and with your drug treatment, if appropriate.

Measuring Your Waistline

It is interesting that the charts don't ask if you are overweight or not. That is largely because being overweight is not a direct risk factor – it seems to work through the other risk factors, like cholesterol and high blood pressure. The higher the blood pressure and the higher the cholesterol, the more likely you are to be overweight, but there are some people who are of normal weight for their height who are still subject to these risk factors.

This does not mean you can look on being overweight as a nuisance, but not something to be much bothered about. If you do bring down your blood pressure and cholesterol levels and stop smoking, you will definitely reduce your risk of a heart attack, but if you remain overweight while you do these things you are still at a slightly increased risk.

The increase in risk that accompanies being overweight applies particularly to men and women with diabetes. If you have adult-onset diabetes, then being overweight carries a considerable extra risk of a heart attack or stroke, even if you are controlling your diabetes, your blood pressure and your cholesterol reasonably well. As mentioned in Chapter Two, being 'apple-shaped' (with the extra weight around your waist, rather than your hips) carries an extra burden of risk, as it means that the extra fat is being laid down around and in the internal organs (including the coronary arteries) rather than under the skin.

What is the best way to know if you are apple-shaped? It is simple. Simply measure yourself around the waist. Men with waist measurements under 94cm and women with waist measurements under 80cm don't need to worry. They are classified as 'non-obese'. Those with waists between 94 and 101cm (for men) and between 80 and 87cm (for women) are in what has been defined as the 'alerting zone'. They should try, with exercise and sensible eating, to lose the extra centimetres. Men with waists above 101cm and women with waists above 87cm need to talk about it to their doctors.

Watching Your Blood Pressure

If you have high blood pressure, you must bring it down to a normal level. Many people are confused about what blood pressure is, and what the two readings they get from their doctor mean, so I have devoted the next chapter to high blood pressure and how it is controlled. All that you need to know here, however, is that your blood pressure is at least as important as your cholesterol level. Once you know you have high blood pressure (your doctor will call it *hypertension*) you must presume that you will have it for the rest of your life. So you must attend regular check-ups (usually once a month, or every three months after it has been brought under control) for it to be measured, and for your drugs to be changed, if necessary. Never assume that because you are feeling well, your blood pressure is normal. Hypertension rarely causes symptoms, and the first sign of the disease may be that heart attack or stroke that you are trying to avoid.

Blood Glucose

This book has already touched several times on diabetes and how it is linked with high cholesterol levels. The best way to tell whether you have diabetes or have a tendency towards developing it is to have your fasting blood glucose level measured. That is, a blood sample is taken in the morning before breakfast, at least 8 and preferably 12 hours after your last food or drink.

Glucose, like cholesterol, is measured in mmol/l in Britain and other European countries, and in mg/dl in North America. For glucose, multiply mmol/l by 18 to get mg/dl. We usually diagnose diabetes if the fasting blood glucose level is above 6.1mmol/l (110mg/dl).

We also recognise a condition called 'impaired glucose tolerance', which can be looked upon as a halfway stage between normality and diabetes. If we suspect you have impaired glucose tolerance, we usually give you a drink of 75g glucose, then take a blood sample two hours later. If it is between 6.7 and 10mmol/l (120 to 180mg/dl), this is considered evidence of poor glucose tolerance.

If you are given a diagnosis of poor glucose tolerance, it is vital you lose any excess weight and stick closely to the healthy eating habits described earlier. If you don't do this you are in danger of developing diabetes later, and you are also raising your heart attack and stroke risk even if you remain free of overt diabetes.

If you have a problem with diabetes or impaired glucose tolerance, you will need to have regular checks on your 'HbA1c'. This is shorthand for the percentage of red blood cells you have circulating in your blood that are coated with glucose. When they are in this state, they cannot carry oxygen around the body efficiently. The higher your HbA1c, the more red cells are affected and the poorer is your blood supply to all vital organs, including your coronary arteries and your brain. So it is best to keep the HbA1c as low as possible, which is done by controlling your blood glucose levels as well as possible. A normal HbA1c in people who haven't got diabetes is around 4 to 5 per cent. In diabetes it can rise well above 10 per cent. We prefer to see it under 7.5 per cent.

Summarising Your Risks

So, you have been told you have a high cholesterol, and maybe some other risk factors, too. You know that:
you mustn't smoke, even one cigarette a day
you must eat healthily
you must be physically active
you must lose any extra pounds (or stones)

you must keep your blood pressure normal
(under 140/90 – see Chapter Eleven)
you must lower your total cholesterol to below 5mmol/l (190mg/dl)
you must reduce your LDL-C to below 3mmol/l (115mg/dl)
if you have diabetes, you must keep your blood glucose and your blood pressure under good control. This means an HbA1c below 7.5 per cent, and a blood pressure below 130/85. Because blood vessels in those with diabetes are more vulnerable to damage by increased pressure, we prefer to lower it more vigorously in people with diabetes than in the rest of the hypertensive population.

How to Change Your Life

All the advice given until now in this book has been very simple to give. It is much harder to TAKE. Psychologists (and general practitioners are nothing if not psychologists) understand very clearly that most people, given the advice to change their lives in a dramatic way (to eat differently, drink less, stop smoking, take exercise and so on), are initially very unwilling to do so.

It is only after careful consideration of all that has been presented to them (and the way in which it has been presented) that people usually start to be willing to change. The process has been described as having five stages – before a person starts thinking, thinking, preparing to change, taking action, and maintaining improvement. Let's take them stage by stage. If you have been asked to read this book by your doctor or by a spouse, relative or friend, you may recognise your own stage in the process.

Before Thinking

This is the stage of being presented with the news that you should alter your ways. You haven't thought about it, and you don't want to think about it. You haven't yet come to terms with the probable long-term risks of continuing with your old lifestyle. You may have thought a bit about changing, but have found it difficult. You may believe, wrongly, that you can't do it, and have become discouraged. You may even have reacted angrily to the pressure put on you by your medical team or your relatives to change, and have stubbornly refused to do so. Unfortunately, some people stick in this stage: they never progress to the next stage. They remain at high risk, and leave themselves much more open to the possibility of an early death from heart attacks and strokes. I've found, as many other doctor colleagues do, that most people understand that lifestyle affects us all – but somehow they relate the message only to others, and not to themselves. I wish I had a pound for every patient who has said 'Why me?' when they eventually have their stroke or serious heart attack, when they had been given the answer to the question repeatedly over the previous years.

The Thinking Stage
In this stage, people have started to think about changing their lives. However, they may stay in the stage of thinking about it for a long time before they actually put their thoughts into practice. They really are no better than those who do not think about changing at all, because they still leave themselves at risk. They are the people who are going to stop smoking 'tomorrow', or just want that last piece of pudding, or will join the gym when the weather gets better. What they need is more motivation, and someone close who can cajole them on to the next stage.

Preparing to Change
The next stage, preparing to change your life, is the one that is most encouraging for most doctors like myself. This is when we – that is, doctor and patient together – start to see results. And with results comes encouragement to go the whole hog into the 'taking action' stage. The 'preparers' have made a diary commitment to start to change, say within the next week. They have drawn up a plan to reduce and then stop their smoking habit, and they plan to start their new eating habits. Just by planning like this, they may well start their scheme early. This is the time when the medical team can move in, in earnest, with help and support from the dietician and the practice nurse, and step up the encouragement from friends and family. That will encourage the person to move on to the stage of real action.

Taking Action
This stage is the one in which people need most help. It is when their resolve is most likely to break down, and they will backslide into the pre-thinking stage. If you are a smoker who wants to stop, be honest

with yourself. How many times have you stopped, felt good about yourself for doing so, then started smoking again within six months? If it is important for the medical and nursing team to help the 'preparer' to progress into the 'active' stage, it is 10 times more important for them to help the preparer sustain the effort.

For example, you cannot consider yourself 'active' if you have merely cut down on your smoking, or have switched brands to one claimed to contain less tar. You are only active if you have stopped completely. If you are overweight, you are only active if you have managed a sustained weight-loss. If you have just cut down on the amount of food, but kept it to chips and fast foods, then you aren't yet active – you need to change the quality as well as the quantity of the food you eat each day.

Maintaining the Improvement

We don't put people into the 'maintenance' category until they have been 'active' for more than six months. It takes that amount of time, for example, for the temptation to return to old habits (smoking, eating too much of the wrong foods, slumping into immobility at the end of the working day) to lessen. But if you last more than six months in the active stage, you will almost certainly find the temptation receding into the past, you will be more confident in yourself, and you may feel more at ease with relatives and friends, who will surely appreciate the effort you have made.

Be honest. In which category can you fairly place yourself? If it is one of the first two, try to move at least into the third. If you are in the third, it should be easy to get into the fourth. If you are in the fourth, do everything you can to seek help from professionals, friends and relatives to keep you in it for at least six months. If you are in the fifth category, give yourself a pat on the back. You deserve it. And you have already done yourself a power of good. Keep up the good work and be happy that your lifestyle change is for the rest of your life. You will enjoy it much better, and for longer, than if you'd stuck in stages one to three.

Chapter Eleven

Blood Pressure

Most people have heard of high blood pressure, and know of someone who has it. You may have it yourself, along with your high cholesterol. But do you know what it is, and what the readings your doctor tells you about mean?

This chapter offers a short explanation of what blood pressure (*hypertension*) is and how we define it. It finishes with a short review of the treatments for high blood pressure, though this is not meant to be comprehensive. If you need to know more about it, please read a copy of my book *Living with High Blood Pressure* (Sheldon Press).

What Blood Pressure Is

The blood pressure that your doctor measures in your arm is the force that drives the blood within the arteries leading from the left side of your heart, taking oxygen from the lungs around the body in its red blood cells. It has two components:

1. The driving force (called the *systolic pressure*) exerted on the blood by the contraction of the main heart muscle, the left ventricle.
2. The resistance to this driving force inside the walls of the arteries, caused by the contraction of the muscle layer in the small arteries. This is the *diastolic pressure*.

The 'blood pressure' is a measure of these two forces. Systolic pressure is always higher than the diastolic pressure, and the blood pressure rises and falls between the two (systolic and diastolic) with each heart beat. The height of the blood pressure is measured in millimetres of mercury (mm Hg). That is the pressure needed to keep a column of mercury at that height above the level of the arm to which the cuff is attached. Most doctors have now switched to a needle-on-a-dial machine, but the tradition of writing the result in equivalent mm Hg remains.

Blood Pressure Readings

In adults, the systolic pressure is usually between 120 and 140mm Hg, and the diastolic between 70 and 90mm Hg. The blood pressure is written as systolic/diastolic, so that a normal pressure would be written, say, as 125/85mm Hg. Normally the blood pressure remains steady through a narrow range. It rises with exercise and under mental or physical stress, but physical and mental relaxation bring it down again. Only when blood pressure remains above the normal (say above 145/90) even after a person has relaxed for several minutes, is it considered abnormally high. Even then, your doctor will ask you to return several times before making a definitive diagnosis.

One of two changes (or both) in the mechanics of normal blood pressure can lead to hypertension:

- the first is the heart beating with too much force, raising the systolic pressure
- the second happens when the muscles around the small arteries in the limbs contract too vigorously, causing them to narrow. This raises the resistance to the flow of blood through them, raising the diastolic pressure.
- In high blood pressure, both pressures are usually raised, although some older people can have a raised systolic pressure with a low diastolic pressure. This is called 'isolated systolic hypertension'. It used to be thought that this type of high blood pressure was less important and less threatening than a combined raised systolic and diastolic pressure, but we now realise that both types should be treated vigorously.

In the past we classified hypertension as being *mild* if the diastolic pressure were between 95 and 104mm Hg, *moderate* if it were between 105 and 115mm Hg, and *severe* when above 115mm Hg. Now we see the risks of high blood pressure as being steadily progressive. The higher it is above the normal, the higher the risk of having a stroke or heart attack.

This steadily increasing risk with a higher pressure is steeper if the cholesterol is also high, if you smoke and/or if you have diabetes. If your diabetes is poorly controlled, the slope is steeper still.

Current medical practice guidelines ask family doctors to try to lower blood pressures that are above 140/90. Not all people in this category need drugs. Lifestyle changes to bring down blood pressure include losing any excess weight, lowering salt intake (most people consume far too much salt), restricting alcohol intake to less than three standard drinks a day (too much alcohol pushes the pressure up, contrary to popular belief that it lowers it). Keeping physically active is also vital to lowering blood pressure. Becoming a couch potato pushes your pressure up, again contrary to popular belief.

Smoking is potentially lethal to people with hypertension, as the damage it inflicts upon the endothelium is multiplied several-fold by the added complication of high blood pressure. So if you have high blood pressure and smoke, you absolutely must stop smoking. Otherwise you are a catastrophe waiting to happen.

Pressure-lowering Drugs

So many trials of the use of anti-hypertensive (pressure-lowering) drugs have shown that they not only bring down high pressures but also lower death rates from heart attacks and strokes, so that their use is now proven beyond any question. So if you remain hypertensive despite the lifestyle changes you have made, you need to take one or another of the current drugs.

Not all antihypertensives are the same, so that it is good to know which one you have been prescribed and which are preferred when you also have a high cholesterol level.

Types of antihypertensive drugs in current common use include diuretics, beta-blockers, calcium antagonists, ACE inhibitors, angiotensin blockers, and alpha-blockers. They have these names because they act on different systems which are part of the overall normal blood pressure control-system in the body. Which one you are prescribed depends on how well they reduce your blood pressure and how well you can tolerate their effects and side-effects.

It is usual practice to start people off with a diuretic and perhaps a beta-blocker. Diuretics may also be combined with an ACE inhibitor or an alpha-blocker. Beta-blockers or ACE inhibitors may be given alongside a calcium antagonist. Your doctor may decide to ring the changes for a few months before settling on the combination that best suits you.

However, if you have a high cholesterol you are more likely to be offered an ACE inhibitor, a calcium antagonist or an alpha-blocker, rather than a beta-blocker or a diuretic, as the latter two types of drugs have been reported as raising levels of LDL-C and TG.

If you want to know more about the drugs you are being prescribed for high blood pressure, don't be afraid to discuss them with your doctor. The modern doctor is happy to explain his or her reasons for prescribing: the days of shrouding prescriptions in medical mystique are long gone.

If you do not have diabetes, your initial blood pressure aim is to get under 140/90mm Hg. Then you can go for a slightly lower pressure. If you have diabetes, then go for under 130/80. It is far more difficult to achieve, but there is plenty of evidence to show that you can hugely reduce your risk of the worst diabetes complications (such as kidney failure, blindness, circulation failure in the feet and hands, heart disease and strokes) if you keep your blood pressure under the strictest control. Your diabetes specialist working with your local general practice team will work hard to help you achieve this goal.

Maintaining a Healthy Blood Pressure

Once you have attained your new, healthier blood pressure, you must accept that you are a hypertensive for life. You will always be on your doctor's list for regular review at the blood pressure clinic. Never think that because you feel well your blood pressure is normal, and that you can stop the tablets or revert to your old lifestyle. It can't be too often repeated that a high blood pressure often gives no symptoms at all, until you have your stroke and/or heart attack. And then it may be too late. One-third of people having their first heart attack or stroke die from it, and another third are considerably disabled by it. It is not worth taking the chance of stopping your treatment yourself, no matter how inconvenient it is to take tablets every day.

Chapter Twelve

Diabetes

If you have diabetes you probably have a high cholesterol level, and you almost certainly have a very high triglyceride level. It is important for you to keep all of these conditions under strict control. This sounds both daunting and dispiriting. It need not be. If you can change your lifestyle in the ways we have mentioned before, with better eating habits, more exercise and just a little self-confidence, you are already more than halfway towards achieving both a near-normal blood glucose and a normal lipid profile.

Types of Diabetes

There are two types of diabetes. The first is Type 1, which usually starts in childhood and needs insulin injections to control it. The second is Type 2, which usually starts in middle life (although, as the population gets fatter, it is increasingly being diagnosed in younger adults). Type 2 is usually treated with lifestyle changes, and sometimes with glucose-lowering drugs that are taken by mouth.

Crucial to the good management of Type 2 diabetes is to lose any excess weight. That can virtually 'cure' the illness in some people. If you wish to read more about managing your diabetes, whether of Type 1 or Type 2, please read 'How to Cope Successfully with Diabetes' also published by Wellhouse. Type 2 diabetes is far more common than Type 1, and is fast expanding: it is estimated that it already affects more than one million people in Britain, and that this figure will double in the next 10 years.

It is enough to state here that good weight control and good blood glucose control almost always bring with them good cholesterol control, because the changes you need to make to bring your glucose under control are the same as those that will bring down cholesterol and triglyceride levels.

Proof that good blood glucose control matters was given by the United Kingdom Prospective Diabetes Study (UKPDS), which compared intensive and ordinary blood glucose control in hundreds of people with Type 2 diabetes. Those under intensive care had an HbA1c of 7 per cent: it was 7.9 per cent in those in the routine care group. (See Chapter Ten to remind yourself about HbA1c.) This apparently small difference in HbA1c made a big difference to the patients' health. Those with the lower HbA1cs had 25 per cent fewer complications with their circulation, and 16 per cent fewer heart attacks over the 10 years in which they were followed up.

So it is really worthwhile, if you have diabetes, to keep your blood glucose level as normal as you can. As mentioned in the last chapter on blood pressure, it is also very beneficial to keep your blood pressure as low as possible. And it is crucial to keep your blood lipids under optimal control.

High TG levels and low HDL-C levels are very common in Type 2 diabetes. If you have this form of diabetes, then your aim is to lower your LDL-C to below 3mmol/l (below 115mg/dl). If you can't achieve this level, your doctor will almost certainly advise you to take a drug that will help you to do so. It may be a fibrate or a statin. The same goals apply if you have impaired glucose tolerance (see Chapter Ten).

This is particularly important for women with diabetes. If you are female and have diabetes, you lose all the natural advantages over men of the same age in protection against heart disease. So you need to be especially careful about your glucose and cholesterol control. The next chapter, therefore, is devoted to women with high cholesterol levels.

Chapter Thirteen

Women and Heart Disease

Ask the general public which section of the population is most likely to have a heart attack, and most people will reply middle-aged men. They don't see heart disease as a risk for women. They are wrong. Coronary heart disease is the most common cause of death among women in North America and Europe, including Britain. It causes more deaths among women, for example, than does breast cancer. In fact, in older people heart disease kills more women than men, because their risk of heart attack rises steeply after the menopause.

Heart attacks also occur in younger women. A quarter of the deaths from a heart attack in women under the age of 65 happen to women under 45 years old. It is true that most women seem to be protected to some degree against heart disease by their hormones before the menopause – but not all of them are. Why some women are so vulnerable has not been made clear until recently.

Part of the fault in not recognising the risk that women run is the medical profession's. All the initial trials and studies of heart attacks and their treatments were conducted in men only – it took years before the first studies in women were started. So we have less factual information about women and their risk of heart disease than we have for men. It took Dr Karen Clarke and her colleagues in Nottingham University to wake the medical world up to its neglect of the risks that women run.

They reported, in 1994, on all people admitted to their hospital in 1989 and 1990 on suspicion that they were having heart attacks. Of those who actually had had full heart attacks, the women took longer than the men to arrive in hospital and were less likely to be admitted to coronary care and to receive the life-saving clot-busting emergency drugs aspirin and streptokinase. They had more severe heart damage, were more ill, and were slightly more likely to die in hospital than the men. Even when they were sent home after recovery from their heart attacks, they were given less follow-up treatment. (For more about aspirin, see Chapter Fourteen.)

Dr Clarke's conclusions that women with heart disease were receiving less than a fair deal were echoed by Dr Paul Wilkinson and his colleagues of the London School of Hygiene and Tropical Medicine. They found lower survival rates for women (70 per cent) than for men (84 per cent) after heart attacks in their hospital.

Why Do Women Not Do So Well?

One reason is that family doctors tended initially not to put chest pain in women down to heart trouble. Another is that because women are on average older than men when they have their first heart attack, they tend to be given less active treatment – because of their age, rather than gender. However, if anything, intensive treatment has better results in older than in younger people with heart attacks. But most of all, what harms women is the ingrained belief that because women have been 'protected' by their hormones during most of their lives, there is less need to bother about high blood cholesterol and triglyceride levels. The logic follows that there should be less need to lower high cholesterol levels in women.

That logic was reinforced by a French finding, many years ago, that the average total cholesterol in 80-year-old Frenchwomen was around 8mmol/l. It was reasoned then that a high cholesterol was good for them, and that the average at 80 was so high because the women who had had lower cholesterol levels had died out before reaching that age.

That logic could not have been more wrong. Frenchwomen have very different eating (and drinking) habits over a lifetime than British women, so that their cholesterol levels are not relevant to women in other countries. The facts in Britain and the United States remain that the higher the blood cholesterol and triglyceride levels in women, the more at risk they are from heart attack and stroke. That risk rises steeply after the menopause, to overtake the corresponding risk in men of the same age, around their late seventies and early eighties.

So it is just as vital for women to take control over their cholesterol and triglyceride levels as it is for men, and even more vital for them to do so as they grow older. If you are female and have a high cholesterol count, do discuss it with your doctor. However, do understand the difference between women and men where the total cholesterol (TC) is concerned. In men a high total cholesterol is virtually always a sign that the LDL-C is raised. This means that you can equate a high total cholesterol level in men directly to their risk of heart attack and stroke.

In women you can't do that. You must measure the different components of the total cholesterol in women. A high total cholesterol in women may mean a high HDL-C. In that case you are not at risk, and do not need to alter your lifestyle or take drugs to lower cholesterol. Only if the rise in total cholesterol is due to a rise in LDL-C or VLDL-C (equivalent to a high TG) should you take action.

The real problem for women arises if their high cholesterol level is accompanied by diabetes, high blood pressure and smoking. The last two chapters dealt with high blood pressure and diabetes. Suffice it to say here that women with high blood pressure, diabetes and a high cholesterol are at an extremely high risk of early heart attacks and strokes, and should take every precaution to make sure that they keep all three under good control.

Smoking is a particular problem for women, and needs an extra mention here. Writing in 2002, I am distressed to learn that more young women than ever in Britain are smoking. They use cigarettes to keep slim or to combat stress, but the habit destroys their complexion, their looks, their lungs and their hearts. It is so difficult for them to stop once they've started. So if you are in the thinking stage (see Chapter Ten about the stages of lifestyle change) about stopping smoking, use these facts about women smokers to help you graduate to the active stage:

Premenopausal smokers have three times the heart attacks of
   non-smoking females of the same age.
Women smoking more than 40 cigarettes a day increase their risk
   of heart attack by a massive 20 times.
If you have diabetes and a high cholesterol level, and smoke,
   you multiply your heart attack risk even more.
Smoking while you are on the contraceptive pill, particularly if
   you are over 35, hugely increases your risk of thrombosis
   (blood clots) in the pelvis, legs, lungs and brain. Many of these
   thromboses are lethal.

Once women have been told that they have heart disease, they are less likely to take up the offer of rehabilitation classes. They are reported to be more depressed, anxious and even to feel guiltier about developing heart disease than men. These feelings must be overcome so that they have at least an equal chance to their male counterparts of a good recovery from their heart attacks.

May I make a special appeal to women readers? Family doctors have been made very much aware of their past shortcomings in their dealings with women who are at risk from, or actually have, heart disease. We are doing our best to put that right. But we need your help. Please recognise that you are at least as much at risk of having a heart attack as your menfolk. Do not ignore any pain in your chest. Never assume, as many women have done in the past, that it is 'indigestion' or a 'hiatus hernia' without first proving that it is not due to angina. Do not smoke, at all. Drink moderately, but preferably not more than three small drinks a day. Never binge-drink – women's livers tolerate binge-drinking less than men's do.

If you have had a heart attack, do take seriously your treatment to prevent further attacks, and accept all the offers of help and advice your doctor, nurse and rehabilitation team give you. Don't feel guilty, and do remain active.

Do have regular health checks, which should include a blood pressure measurement and blood tests for cholesterol, triglycerides and glucose, so that you know your risk and know what you can do to reduce it. Do try to keep to a normal weight, neither too fat nor too thin. If you are in the menopause and beyond, discuss the possibility of hormone replacement therapy with your doctor. The decision to go on HRT depends on many factors which are individual to each woman, so that this is not the place to give advice either way on it. But if you have your doctor's blessing on it, it could help your heart and circulation.

Chapter Fourteen

Aspirin and Other Drugs

Doctors who read both the *Lancet* and the *British Medical Journal* were justifiably puzzled on January 12, 2002. The *Lancet* ran a leading article entitled 'No reduction in cardiovascular risk [i.e. the risk of stroke and heart attack] with NSAIDs – including aspirin?' The *British Medical Journal* (*BMJ*) of the same day published a paper confirming not only that aspirin reduces the risk of heart attacks and strokes in susceptible people, but even proposed that doctors could extend the range of patients who would benefit from being given aspirin.

What were we to believe? Here is another bold statement, this time from the *Clinician's Manual on Total Risk Management* published by Science Press in London, a booklet intended to help in the training of young hospital doctors. Its authors, all well-known cardiologists, wrote that aspirin 'should be administered to virtually all patients with coronary or other atherosclerotic disease'. They include in this definition all patients after myocardial infarction (heart attack), and those with manifestations of coronary disease such as angina. It should also be given, they write, to people with hypertension.

Aspirin for High Cholesterol?

Should aspirin also be given to people with only one of the trio of risk factors – a high cholesterol?

Let us start from the basic premise that an uncontrolled and constantly high blood total cholesterol level will lead eventually to heart disease and stroke, because of the damage it does to the arteries in the heart and brain. That leads to the propensity of blood to clot in an area of such damage, so that it is necessary not just to lower the cholesterol level, but also to try to prevent the mechanism that leads to the clot. The best way we know how to do that is to prescribe a small dose of aspirin every day. The aspirin treatment does certainly reduce heart attacks and stroke rates in people at high risk of them.

So why do the *BMJ* and *Lancet* differ on its use? The *BMJ* looked at the results of 287 studies involving 138,000 patients given aspirin or a similar agent compared with 'controls' (who did not receive the drugs), and 77,000 in trials comparing aspirin and one of the other drugs. The analysis is too complex to be described here, but the results were clear, especially because the numbers are so large.

The patients in the studies were all at seriously high risk of dying from a heart attack or stroke. They were given the aspirin or other drug to see if they could avoid these disasters. Success was measured by comparing the numbers of serious heart or brain 'events' during the follow-up period.

On average, in those who had had a previous heart attack, aspirin led to 36 fewer serious events for every 1,000 people treated for two years. There were 38 per 1,000 fewer events within the next month among people who started treatment during a heart attack. There were 36 fewer heart attacks and strokes in the following two years per 1,000 people who had had previous strokes, and 9 fewer serious events in the following three weeks per 1,000 people who started treatment during a stroke. The benefits of reduction in such events far outweighed the small extra risk of bleeding caused by the aspirin.

The other drugs with which aspirin was compared were clopidogrel (an anti-platelet agent with aspirin-like properties but theoretically with less risk of irritating the stomach), and dipyridamole, a blood vessel-widening agent. Whether or not you can be prescribed clopidogrel or dipyridamole depends on your doctor's assessment and practice. However, the *BMJ* article was in no doubt that aspirin in a dose of 75mg to 150mg daily (a quarter to a half of the standard 300-mg aspirin tablet) should be given to anyone with more than a 2 per cent risk of having a heart attack or a stroke within the next year. This includes people with the recognised risk factors but who are still apparently well, who do not have angina and have not had a heart attack or stroke.

Most people with a high cholesterol level are around this level of risk. If they also have diabetes, high blood pressure or smoke, their risk is likely to be well above that level. So if you are in this category, you should probably take half an aspirin a day, to lower your risk.

Clopidogrel is usually reserved for people who cannot tolerate aspirin. The extra benefit of dipyridamole is doubtful. People undergoing coronary balloon surgery or bypass surgery, or who are in a very severe angina attack, who are at immediate risk of a heart attack, may also be offered treatment with a 'glycoprotein IIb/IIIa antagonist' which is a very powerful anti-clotting agent.

So why did the *Lancet* disagree with the *BMJ*? The study it published was performed by Professor Wayne Ray, of the Vanderbilt University School of Medicine, Nashville, Tennessee. Professor Ray and his colleagues had followed more than 180,000 users of 'non-aspirin-non-steroidal anti-inflammatory drugs' (NANSAIDs) and a similar number of non-users of these drugs, to note how many were admitted to hospital for, or died from, coronary disease. The study ran from January 1 1987 and ended on December 31 1998.

NANSAIDs are drugs designed to act like aspirin in reducing inflammation, fever and pain, but in theory with less irritant action on the stomach. They are now in popular use as ibuprofen, naproxen and indomethacin: most people will recognise these names from products on pharmacy shelves.

The Tennessee study failed to find any protective effect of any of the NANSAIDs. There were just as many heart attacks among the users as among the non-users of NANSAIDs. The authors concluded that NANSAIDs should not be used to prevent heart attacks or strokes.

However, aspirin did not feature in the Tennessee study. So why did the *Lancet* cast doubt on the value of aspirin for people at risk of a coronary? The journal asked Dr John Cleland, of the University of Hull, to comment on the Tennessee work. He cast doubt on the results of many of the trials analysed, stating that too many of them had contained too few patients, and that some small trials may not have been published because they did not have positive results.

The controversy will continue. My own feeling is that a once-a-day aspirin (75mg) will harm very few people, and the evidence so far seems to indicate that it should help more by putting off their impending stroke or heart attack. I have absolutely no doubt (nor does Dr Cleland) that there is good evidence for taking aspirin for at least six weeks after a heart attack. Where we tend to differ is what to do after that. I am looking forward to Dr Cleland's own study, in which he and many others are comparing the effects of aspirin, clopidogrel and warfarin in people who are in heart failure.

Dr Cleland feels, too, that the aspirin treatment may have caused us to neglect to prescribe other 'better proven and apparently more effective therapies, such as angiotensin-converting enzyme inhibitors (ACE inhibitors), beta-blockers and statins, for patients with or at high risk of cardiovascular disease'. With that I do wholly agree.

We have described in detail the benefits of statins, and no more needs be written here about them. Beta-blockers have been shown to reduce deaths from heart attacks when given immediately after the attack and for several months afterwards. So everyone who can tolerate beta-blockers (a few people, such as those with asthma, cannot) should be given them after a heart attack or severe angina attack. If they cannot tolerate a beta-blocker, then a 'long-acting' calcium antagonist drug (see Chapter Eleven for the types of drug used in high blood pressure) should be given instead.

ACE inhibitors (also see Chapter Eleven) are given when people who have had heart attacks have enough damage to their heart muscle to reduce its efficiency to around 40 per cent of normal. This is defined as heart failure, and people with it are usually breathless at the slightest exertion. Trials have shown that ACE inhibitors improve the heart's efficacy, at the same time improving the person's quality of life, so they are worthwhile. ACE inhibitors are also useful in preventing deterioration of the kidneys in diabetes.

A last group of drugs that must be considered for anyone at high risk of a heart attack are the 'anticoagulants'. The best known of these is warfarin, mainly because it has been publicised as the human version of rat poison. Warfarin must be given in carefully chosen doses, according to how long it takes for a sample of the person's blood to clot. So people prescribed warfarin must have very frequent blood tests to make sure that they are on the right dose. Too little and the blood clots too easily. Too large a dose and the person may start to bleed spontaneously internally. Most family doctors now have a warfarin clinic, which their patients attend at least weekly (and sometimes more often) to make sure their bleeding is under optimal control.

Warfarin is given to people with several problems after, say, a heart attack. Some, for example, have been left with an abnormal area of heart muscle that does not contract in tune with the rest of the heart.

Others have an irregular heartbeat known as *atrial fibrillation*, which can cause a clot to form within one of the upper chambers of the heart (the atrium). It is also given to people who have had heart valves replaced, to stop clots forming on them, and to people who have had previous thromboses.

Chapter Note

Chapter Two   [1]A G Shaper and colleagues, *Journal of
Epidemiology and Community Health* 1985,
volume 39, pages 197-209

Glossary

Atheroma Fatty porridge-like deposits in the walls of arteries, that are the sites of thromboses and haemorrhages, leading to heart attacks and strokes.

Atherosclerosis The disease process that produces deposits of atheroma in arteries.

Cholesterol The group name for many fatty substances found in the blood and tissues.

Fibrates A group of drugs used mainly to treat hypertriglyceridaemia (high VLDL), but may also be a second choice against high LDL.

Hyperglycaemia High blood sugar levels, found in diabetes.

Hyperlipidaemia Excessively high levels of lipids (fats) in the blood. This encompasses hypercholesterolaemia, high total cholesterol levels.

Hypertension High blood pressure.

Lipids The medical term for fats.

Lipoproteins Compounds of fats and proteins used by the body for many processes, and transported throughout the body combined with cholesterol. Subdivided into classes according to their density - such as high density (HDL), low density (LDL) and very low density (VLDL).

HDL: The type of lipoprotein that carries fats out of blood vessel walls, thereby reducing atheroma.

LDL: A type of lipoprotein that encourages fats to be deposited into blood vessel walls, thereby increasing atheroma.

VLDL: A type of lipoprotein usually linked to triglyceride, and like LDL linked to increasing atheroma.

Statins A group of drugs used to treat hyperlipidaemia, mainly to lower high LDL.

Triglyceride A complex of carbohydrate and fats, high levels of which are found in the blood in diabetes and obesity. As with LDL and VLDL, rising triglyceride levels are linked to atheroma.

Index

Other titles available in the

HOW TO COPE
SUCCESSFULLY WITH series...

HOW TO COPE SUCCESSFULLY WITH

DIVERTICULITIS

Dr Joan McClelland

Diverticulitis is a Cinderella disorder. It is very common, can be dangerous and there are rapidly increasing numbers of sufferers. We stand a more than 50 per cent chance of suffering from diverticulitis before we reach the age of 60. Dr Joan McClelland describes in her easily accessible style the symptoms, different types of diverticulitis, complications and various treatments including alternative and herbal remedies. This book also covers the psychological aspects of diverticulitis and the benefits of exercise and diet.

ISBN: 1-903784-00-X   128pp

HOW TO COPE SUCCESSFULLY WITH

ANXIETY AND DEPRESSION

Beth MacEoin

We live in stressful times and have to cope on a daily basis with a variety of different pressures. These can include financial worries, emotional stresses, bereavement, break-up of relationships and insecurity at work. When feeling well and resilient we are able to cope with a wide range of these stressful situations. It is when we become mentally and emotionally overloaded at a vulnerable time in our lives that we can suffer from symptoms of anxiety or depression. Beth MacEoin describes in her easily accessible style the various symptoms and suggests a wide range of practical measures to provide positive support.

ISBN: 1-903784-03-4   128pp

YOUR LIFESTYLE DIET

Karen Sullivan

A healthy diet is more than just balancing food intake, it involves eating foods that promote rather than endanger health. What are the elements of a healthy balanced diet? How do we identify which are good fats, bad fats and essential fats? What problems can be caused by sugar in our diet? What are the different types of sugars found in our diet and which are healthy? What should we drink and what should we avoid drinking? What essential supplements do we need? The answers to these questions and many more are contained in Your Lifestyle Diet.

ISBN: 1-903784-04-2   128pp

MENOPAUSE

Dr Joan McClelland

The menopause is an event to welcome, a stimulating new chapter in your life. You can say goodbye to period pains, water retention, PMS together with a host of psychological problems including irritability, depression and chronic tension. The menopause is a vantage point from which to take stock, reviewing your earlier life and looking ahead to new interests, deepening relationships and fresh goals. You are entering an important and fascinating time in your life and to get the best out of it you need to work in harmony with nature, this book aims to help you achieve this aim.

ISBN: 1-903784-05-0   128pp

HOW TO COPE SUCCESSFULLY WITH

DIABETES

Dr Tom Smith

If there was ever a role model for people with diabetes, insulin-dependent or otherwise, Sir Stephen Redgrave is it. Few people with diabetes aspire to his Olympic gold medal heights but everyone can take heart from the way he put his body through the most rigorous training and still kept good control of his diabetes. The main aim of this book is to achieve a good quality of life despite the health hiccup of diabetes. This book describes all aspects of the healthy lifestyle that every person with diabetes needs to follow, it is positive and optimistic to give people with diabetes a sense that they can shape their own future.

ISBN: 1-903784-02-6   128pp

HOW TO COPE SUCCESSFULLY WITH

THYROID PROBLEMS

Dr Tom Smith

The thyroid is not a subject that immediately springs to mind when we chat socially about our health. We marvel how some people have boundless energy while others are always tired and weary. There are nervous, anxious, agitated people who can never sit still. It is easy to assume that people differ in these ways because of their characters or lifestyle but a substantial number have developed these characteristics through no fault of their own. These are the sufferers from thyroid problems. Do Tom Smith describes in his easily accessible style the symptoms, different types of thyroid problems, complications and the various treatments available today.

ISBN: 1-903784-01-8   128pp

HOW TO COPE SUCCESSFULLY WITH

HIGH BLOOD PRESSURE

Dr Duncan Dymond

Blood Pressure is not a disease, everyone has a pressure, we need it to keep us upright and alive. Your blood pressure varies depending on your level of physical and mental stress. In this easily accessible book Dr Dymond describes what high blood pressure is, the symptoms, various medications available, side effects and possible complications. The tests and investigations for high blood pressure are explained together with treatments and suggestions for changes to lifestyle and diet.

ISBN: 1-903784-07-7   128pp

HOW TO COPE SUCCESSFULLY WITH

PANIC ATTACKS

Karen Sullivan

Panic attacks are a much more common problem than is generally realised an affect a large proportion of the population. They can manifest themselves in many ways including agoraphobia, anticipatory anxiety, separation anxiety, school or work phobia. This book explains what Panic Attacks are, the causes, how panic affects daily life and the associated disorders. Conventional treatments together with their side effects are explained and alternative remedies including acupuncture, homoeopathy, reflexology, massage are covered. Karen Sullivan gives reassuring short term measures to help deal with an attack and, together with other advice, Top Ten Tips to help cope in the longer term.

ISBN: 1-903784-08-5   128pp

HOW TO COPE SUCCESSFULLY WITH

IRRITABLE BOWEL SYNDROME

Richard Emerson

Irritable Bowel Syndrome is a complex problem with both physical and psychological symptoms. The aim of this book is to set out clearly and concisely these symptoms and the various treatments now available – conventional, complementary and alternative. Ths should enable sufferers to improve their lifestyle and either cure or manage their Irritable Bowel Syndrome.

ISBN: 1-903784-06-9   128pp